CHINESE MEDICINE

MANFRED PORKERT, M. D.,
WITH DR. CHRISTIAN ULLMANN

TRANSLATED AND ADAPTED BY
Mark Howson

AN OWL BOOK
HENRY HOLT AND COMPANY
NEW YORK

Henry Holt and Company, Inc.
Publishers since 1866
115 West 18th Street
New York, New York 10011

Henry Holt® is a registered trademark
of Henry Holt and Company, Inc.

Library of Congress Cataloging-in-Publication Data
Howson, Mark.
Chinese medicine / Manfred Porkert, with Christian Ullmann;
translated and adapted by Mark Howson. — 1st Owl book ed.
p.   cm.
Reprint. Originally published: New York : Morrow, c 1988.
"An Owl book."
Includes bibliographical references.
1. Medicine, Chinese. I. Ullmann, Christian.
II. Porkert, Manfred. Chinesiche Medizin. III. Title.
[R602.H68   1990]   89-26792
610'.951—dc20   CIP

ISBN 0-8050-1277-X

Henry Holt books are available for special promotion's
and premiums. For details contact: Director, Special Markets.

First published in the United States in hardcover in 1988 by
William Morrow and Company, Inc.
First Owl Book Edition—1990

Designed by Marie-Hélène Fredrickes

Printed in the United States of America
All first editions are printed on acid-free paper.∞

3   5   7   9   10   8   6   4   2

FOREWORD

IN spite of all our best intentions, Western science has still not adequately come to terms with the phenomenon of Chinese culture. It has, of course, been a commonplace for some time that the Chinese discovered the compass, movable type, and the firing of porcelain, but we have not really considered these useful inventions to be well and truly "discovered" until such time as they became available to our ancestors in the West. And, what is more important, we have managed to perceive very few of these outstanding Chinese discoveries in the context of a civilization that has been developing for over two thousand years. And as far as the compass, the printing press, and porcelain are concerned, there is really a great deal more to be considered than the simple matter of historical priority.

In order to discover what is authentically Chinese about printing or porcelain, we should by no means limit ourselves to the conventional Western technical vocabulary and ideational categories in discussing them. And in order to find out all about Chinese medicinal plants or other traditional *materia medica,* it would not be enough just to tramp the Chinese countryside with test tubes and collecting box in order to subject this haphazardly assembled collection of traditional Chinese remedies to the rigorously evolved analytic scrutiny of Western pharmacology. At best, this is simply a way of discovering which of these Chinese remedies are suitable candidates for inclusion in the Western pharmacopeia (even if they have previously been quite unknown to medicine outside East Asia). This procedure, however rigorous, however exhaustive, really tells us nothing about Chinese medicine as such.

Only when we have managed to understand the cultural background and the intellectual advances that produced these remarkable examples of human creativity so very many years before they appeared in Europe will we begin to grasp exactly what the difference might have been

6   between a "Chinese" and a "European" compass, for example. Apart from its physical properties, there are also certain cultural hallmarks by which we can distinguish this unprepossessing iron needle as "Chinese." And only when we have forgotten about chemical analysis will we understand those particular qualities that have earned certain herbs and plants their place in traditional Chinese medicine. To this end we must be consciously willing to abandon our usual criteria and immerse ourselves in the Chinese way of thinking and the Chinese way of looking at the world.

Still, without some knowledge of Chinese, this is no easy task, and even sinologists sometimes have difficulty in laying their hands on certain texts that are essential to any comprehensive understanding or rational reconstruction of Chinese science. Some of the "classics" of traditional Chinese medicine have been out of print for a good eight hundred years, and the existing translations all suffer from various linguistic deficiencies. Thus we must account it an extraordinary piece of good fortune that Mao Zedong decreed an end to the long decadence and decline of traditional Chinese medicine, and consequently during the 1950s virtually the entire canon of Chinese medical literature was reissued in scrupulously prepared new editions. These volumes, once I had systematically gathered them all together, became the basis of my twenty-year study of Chinese medicine; my efforts were then devoted to the compilation of a standard glossary of terms in four Western languages (Latin, French, German, and English) that would correspond to the specialized terminology of the original texts. I was also engaged in a thorough examination of the theoretical principles of Chinese medicine, and once this enterprise seemed to be on a firm enough footing, I ventured into such specialized areas as Chinese diagnostic technique and pharmacology, which became the subjects of several textbooks and numerous technical articles. A series of lecture courses enabled medical students to round out their Western medical education with a brief exposure to Chinese traditional medicine, and all this finally led to the establishment of an organization called Societas Medicinae Sinensis.

My coauthor on this book, Christian Ullmann, has primarily concerned himself with the problems in the history of science that are presented by this subject and with an attempt at the rational reconstruction of the formal organization of a non-Western scientific system. In this book we attempt to present the theory and the practice of traditional Chinese medicine in a way that is both comprehensive and comprehensible to the general reader; accordingly, we have tried to exercise special care over the sections in which the reader is first introduced to the Chinese way of thinking about healing and medicine. There are also a great many other aspects of Chinese science, not specifically concerned with medicine, that are nevertheless well worth explaining in this connection. Taken together, they represent the most elaborate and comprehensive scientific system to have developed outside the Western world (by which we mean, to be formulated originally in a non–Indo-European language).

In this book we shall attempt, as far as possible, to examine the Chinese scientific outlook from within; thus we will naturally be concerned not just with medicine but also with everything that touches the life of the individual and of men and women in society and the very workings of the universe itself.

—MANFRED PORKERT

Contents

CONTENTS

CHINESE
MEDICINE

I

CHINESE AND WESTERN MEDICINE

Medicine's Unsolved Problems

JUST a century ago medical science was held spellbound by a dazzling vision of the future. A country doctor named Robert Koch was the first to demonstrate that infectious diseases, which in those days took a greater toll of lives than all of Europe's wars, were actually caused by living microorganisms. Koch isolated the anthrax bacillus in 1876, the bacteria that cause tuberculosis and anthrax a few years later; he also discovered the means of combating these deadly diseases and bringing them under control. Koch was acclaimed as the founder of modern bacteriology, and almost overnight the possibility that all of these ancient scourges of humanity could be eliminated seemed almost within reach; the idea of a life without sickness no longer seemed like a utopian dream. "Medical science received so much credit in the press that it took on a whole new significance in human culture."[1]

Today, over a century later, we must acknowledge that this dream has come true. Smallpox and the plague have been virtually eradicated all over the world, and such frightful epidemic diseases as cholera, typhoid fever, poliomyelitis, diphtheria, and typhus are now completely under control in those countries that enjoy a reasonable standard of sanitation and medical care. Isolation wards, which at one time not so very long ago were an essential part of every hospital, are now largely retained for reasons of prudence rather than by necessity. Perhaps the most eloquent tribute to the effectiveness of modern Western medicine can be found in public-health statistics. Infant mortality in West Germany has been reduced from 226 per thousand live births in 1900 to less than thirteen per thousand today. The annual death rate in Germany has fallen from 22 per ten thousand inhabitants to 12, and adult life expectancy has risen remarkably, from forty-five to seventy-five years.

But in spite of all these impressive statistics, we are compelled to admit that our great-grandparents' expectations that science would banish not

16   only infectious disease but also illness itself from our lives have been cruelly disappointed. The first goal has largely been achieved (hence the changes in the statistics just cited) but not the second; science has prolonged our lives, but the ideal of health still remains elusive. Numerous "new" diseases have risen to take the place of old ones that doctors have learned to deal with and medical science has thoroughly investigated, and against these, Western medicine is powerless—or there is not all that much that can be done. "In many cases medical science prevents the patient from dying," writes Dr. Arthur Jores of Hamburg, in a work titled *Medicine in the Crisis of Our Times*, "without restoring him to health. It is thus a primary cause of chronic illness."[2] And historian of science Theodor Meyer-Steineg writes: "The theater of operations in the doctors' battle against death has since completely shifted. Cancer and disorders of the cardiovascular system have replaced the infectious diseases as the chief causes of death."[3] This battle has grown increasingly costly as well, the terrain increasingly mysterious and puzzling to the combatants, and—if our interpretation of certain indices is correct—the tide of battle actually seems to be turning against us. Life expectancy has actually declined in certain age groups of the elderly population, and demographers have already posed the troubling question of whether "we are on the verge of a downward trend in life expectancy."[4]

A danger signal like this should not be ignored. Never before in history have so much effort and so much money been expended on medical care; nevertheless, there appears to be a constant number of patients whose suffering medical science has been virtually powerless to alleviate. Heidelberg physiologist Hans Schaefer even feels that "there cannot be a significant diagnosis in the case of a considerable minority of patients, perhaps even the majority."[5] Arthur Jores refers to a study of the patients treated by group medical practices in Hamburg, fully half of whom were classified as chronically ill. A further 30 to 40 percent were said to be suffering from "neurotic ailments," which leaves us with a mere 10 to 20 percent of patients whose illnesses respond "correctly" to the standard medical procedure. Modern medicine, as Jores puts it, "in comparison to the healing arts of the old-fashioned general practitioner, primarily benefits those who hardly ever get sick."[6]

And these findings appear in an even more unflattering light when we observe that by no means do all sick people become "patients." In fact, as sociologist Christof Helberger has pointed out, "studies show that between half and two thirds of physical complaints do not result in a visit to a doctor's office. And these complaints are not necessarily trivial in nature—one need only consult the statistics on untreated illnesses and the early stages of chronic disease."[7] On the other hand, surveys of jobholders reveal that fewer than 10 percent of respondents consider themselves really to be healthy, whereas about 60 percent consider themselves to be "in need of medical care to some extent."[8] In opinion samplings (of the general population) more than 40 percent of respondents felt that the state of their general health "could be better."[9]

These various indications of the inadequate state of health of a great many of our compatriots (and the corresponding inadequacies of Western medical science) might suggest any number of conclusions, all of them perfectly appropriate. But it is not our purpose here to frame an indictment of Western medicine; if we are to have a rational medical science at all, then there can be no conceivable alternative. We feel it is much more important to focus our attention on a single disquieting development—or rather a double one, the twofold sense of alienation that has arisen not only between patient and doctor but also between the practicing physician and medical science itself.

THE DOCTOR'S DILEMMA

The task of the practicing physician is to help restore his patients to health, and the means at his disposal are provided by medical science, which means that he bears a responsibility to both. But how is he supposed to proceed with a patient who is suffering from an illness that medical science has still not provided him with the proper procedure for? And what is he expected to do when the most scrupulous diagnosis doesn't yield any positive results? In such cases the doctor can only pursue his task of healing by prescientific means, perhaps guided by certain experiential standards, which is frequently a fairly risky undertaking for the patient, since the success of the treatment is even farther from being guaranteed than in the case of those procedures that are fully sanctioned by medical science. And the risk run by the physician is in certain ways just as great, since when a treatment proves unsuccessful, the patient is much more likely to conclude that he has fallen into the hands of an incompetent doctor than he is to lose his faith in medical science. The doctor must also reckon with the peculiar capriciousness of medical science, which cannot provide him with the means to cure his patients but still condemns as "unscientific" any course of treatment it has not expressly sanctioned.

One way for the doctor to deal with these complaints is to trivialize

18   them, a course of action that medical science will be much more willing to endorse than the use of unorthodox or unconventional procedures. This has been the fate of patients with "neurotic" or "psychosomatic" complaints for some time now—30 to 40 percent of all patients, according to Arthur Jores's findings. "They were the unacknowledged stepchildren of medicine," he writes, "who were dismissed for the most part as malingerers and treated with general contempt."[10] Perhaps no less consequential for the patients involved is the widespread opinion among doctors that such complaints are not "well-defined, serious illnesses,"[11] and by "serious" is meant "life-threatening." But, as we have already mentioned, the "serious" illnesses have largely lost their terrors for us today, and not simply because they are not all that common and because medical science now has excellent means of coping with them. In addition, the patient is removed from his social milieu the moment the disease is diagnosed and returns only after he has completely recovered. By contrast, someone who is suffering from a less "serious" complaint is expected to carry on as usual with his job, and family and other social obligations, even though his doctor is frequently unable to do anything to relieve his suffering. Besides the illness itself, there is the danger of misunderstanding by the patient's friends and associates, his own growing anxiety about not being able to keep working, which in turn may give rise to conflict in the workplace, the "flight" into alcoholism . . . a continuing downward spiral. Today the genuinely serious illnesses are not so much those that are "life-threatening" but those that threaten the individual's entire existence.

THE INCURABLE PATIENT

Patients whose doctors can do nothing to help them still have various alternatives open to them. All sorts of attempts have been made to provide the victims of these intractable illnesses with social compensations of some kind, even with enhanced social status—as in the case of ulcer sufferers and the other victims of "executive stress" of the 1950s. (Today this tendency has given way to the more democratic "midlife crisis," in which anyone can participate as soon as he or she reaches thirty-five.) Others may feel that their sufferings will be easier to bear in the company of their fellow sufferers—the principle on which Alcoholics Anonymous is based—and so they seek each other out and form groups and associations. With certain illnesses, encounter-group therapy has been shown to be more effective than individual treatment, though this does not necessarily rule out individual initiative of the sort that resulted in an ad in a newspaper personals column inserted by "Good-looking Guy, 29, 6', thin, athletic" and afflicted with psoriasis who was seeking a "woman or girl 18 or over with aforementioned problem, as lover & much, much more."[12]

Every patient whose doctor has, despite his best efforts, been unable to help him will eventually seek a second opinion (at the very least) and make the rounds of the specialists. He may even check into a diagnostic clinic for a "good going-over," but like many patients, he may well end up with a series of fresh disappointments to add to his original woes. At long last he may discover what he is not suffering from, but he will still have no idea what is really the matter with him. "Modern medicine has long since become a vast galaxy unto itself, through which the sick man wanders in hopeless confusion—and in which, with the increase of specialization, the ranks of competent advisers and councillors are inexorably growing thinner." So writes internist Thure von Uexküll, one of Europe's most prominent practitioners in the field of psychosomatic medicine. He continues, "Specialists are only experts in their own—restricted—fields, and this is not only regrettable but even dangerous. The way that medicine is taught, each organ becomes the basis of a separate subject, but diseases rarely confine themselves to a single organ of the body. Thus, one may say without exaggeration that a patient who consults one of these highly specialized physicians will often receive not only inadequate medical care but the wrong treatment altogether."[13]

THE CURRENT LIMITS OF MEDICAL KNOWLEDGE

The term *iatrogenic*[14] was coined to describe any illness that is inadvertently caused by a physician or by the incorrect administration of medical treatment. This is by no means the same thing as *malpractice,* though the terms are often used interchangeably in everyday language, since malpractice can occur only when a doctor acts negligently or is simply ignorant of the accepted medical procedure. But is it accurate to speak of malpractice in a case where there is *no* standard procedure? And should the doctor refuse to treat such a case, on the strength of the argument that the state of medical knowledge is not sufficiently advanced and the risk to the patient would accordingly be too great? But if the success of such treatments is going to be judged in the public forum according to the same moral and legal standards that are used to distinguish genuine malpractice, then a doctor can hardly be blamed if he refuses even to consider such a course and sends his patient on to his next port of call in the uncharted galaxy of modern medicine. (In this way he is only

20   protecting himself from the kind of social and financial calamity that may threaten his own existence.)

Nevertheless, the medical community itself is not entirely blameless in this connection, since during the previous heroic age of its most impressive successes it did much to establish the image of medicine as a perfect science, by definition, with no new or unknown diseases beyond its ken. Medical science has managed to keep this reputation more or less intact (though somewhat tarnished and corroded where it has come into contact with reality). But what sort of mistakes could be made in the service of perfect science—other than "human error," of course, which is to say, malpractice? Certainly modern medicine would be better served by presenting the public with a realistic idea of its own limitations than by beguiling it with dream-images of perfection.

Arthur Jores has even discerned "considerable gaps in present-day medical science" and asks if "no more than further research will be required to fill them." The answer he gives is rather pessimistic: "The enormous sums that have been spent on medical research worldwide make it seem very unlikely. Does it not seem more likely, in fact, that there has been some fundamental oversight? And it is precisely our complete lack of knowledge of the fundamental causes of the diseases that assail modern man that is the most perplexing thing of all."[15] Clearly medical science is in a difficult position here. Unlike most other sciences, whose relative progress or lack thereof is not really all that important to us, the unsolved problems of modern medical science will continue to cause a great deal of human suffering, and suffering has necessarily been the primary focus of medical research thus far—for, as Jores observes, "Guided by a shrewd instinct, the research facilities simply pounced on those diseases that would prove the most responsive to the methods of medical science."[16]

SIGNS OF CRISIS?

But for the sort of patients that we are concerned with here, this just means that they should not expect much help from Western medicine. And thus they can hardly be blamed for choosing the third (and increasingly popular) response when academic medicine fails to meet their needs, and placing their bets on some less conventional brand of medicine or on the ministrations of a faith healer or some other practitioner outside the realm of medicine altogether. This is hardly a development that practicing physicians can remain indifferent to. They must first decide if they wish to accompany their patients in this flight into the unorthodox (in spite of all the warnings of medical science) or to resign themselves to their loss. In this case, however, they may still opt for a kind of career change, though without abandoning orthodox medicine.

In addition to the standard fields of specialization (so much deplored by Dr. Thure von Uexküll) based on organs and anatomical systems, doctors are beginning, in a cautious, career-minded way, to take up specialties based on the various spheres of their patients' ordinary lives—occupational health and safety, family medicine, sports medicine, and others. Thus the distinction between preventive and curative medicine is becoming increasingly sharp. Doctors are now serving as consultants on automotive and other "bionomic" engineering projects and on the rational design of factory ventilation systems. These accomplishments—as significant as they might be—will only benefit the "patient" indirectly, and the doctor will have to find his professional satisfaction in a projected long-term improvement in the health and mortality statistics. (On the other hand, the doctor still finds himself fighting a perpetual holding action in which—with vaccination, for example—he is trying to prevent the outbreak of disease at the same time that he is trying to treat it.)

Breaking the Language Barrier

COULD Arthur Jores be right in suggesting that Western medicine has reached its present impasse because of some "fundamental oversight," some flaw in the original blueprint that might actually prevent the great edifice of Western medicine from reaching completion? This seemingly hopeless situation was anticipated by American linguist Benjamin Lee Whorf almost fifty years ago; he was the first to suggest that the use of technical language might turn out to be more of a hindrance than an aid to scientific progress, and he further suggested that a thorough examination of the linguistic underpinnings of modern thought was very much in order. "We cut nature up," he wrote, "organize it into concepts, and ascribe significances as we do, largely because we are parties to an agreement to organize it in this way—an agreement that holds throughout our speech community and is codified in the patterns of our language. The agreement is, of course, an implicit and unstated one, BUT ITS TERMS ARE ABSOLUTELY OBLIGATORY; we cannot talk at all except by subscribing to the organization and classification of data which the agreement decrees."[17]

Through an extensive study of American Indian languages, Whorf found his way into a new world—one that is quite alien to any native speaker of an Indo-European language. He came to the conclusion that the language we speak largely predetermines the way in which "the personality not only communicates, but also analyzes nature, notices or neglects types of relationship and phenomena, channels his reasoning, and builds the house of his consciousness."[18] *And thus language creates for a community of scientists a finite reservoir of potential solutions to problems, and when these are exhausted, scientific progress is no longer possible.* Or, as Whorf puts it, "It needs but half an eye to see in these latter days that science, the Grand Revelator of modern Western culture, has reached, without having intended to, a frontier. Either it must bury its dead, close

24 its ranks, and go forward into a landscape of increasing strangeness, replete with things shocking to a culture-trammeled understanding, or it must become, in Claude Houghton's expressive phrase, the plagiarist of its own past. The frontier was foreseen in principle very long ago, and given a name that has descended to our day clouded with myth. That name is Babel."[19]

THE CONFUSION OF TONGUES IN MEDICINE

And in the meantime, the spate of fresh medical literature that rolls off the presses every day has become so overwhelming that it requires the most sophisticated data-processing equipment just to keep up with it. Very few countries can afford to set up and maintain such elaborate information retrieval systems, and even when a doctor has access to all this material, it is scarcely possible for him to keep up with new developments in his own very narrow field of interest. The transmission of information across the frontiers of the various medical specialties is even more of a problem, even though the parties involved—surgeons and radiologists, for instance—might be concerned with treatment of the same disease.

Another source of linguistic confusion is the separate and thus far uncoordinated development of medical technology across national boundaries. In many countries this is closely associated with national prestige, another useful index of the superiority of one's own social system over one's neighbor's. Consequently these research projects are carried on in splendid isolation and at great cost in human and material resources. The data that finally emerge from these projects cannot be usefully compared, nor can the experiments be replicated at other research facilities. A good example of this is the current research (which has been going on for some time now) on high-speed neutron beams as a treatment for cancer. Everyone has his own equipment and his own particular system, and since the Americans and the British were the first to report some therapeutic benefit for this technique, the French, Germans, Japanese, Italians, et al. were obliged to report that these results could only be accepted with significant reservations—in light of their own ongoing research—or not at all. The different technical setups involved have introduced variables into the reported data, and the resulting quantitative problems are still being ironed out at a series of international conferences.

But why does the progress of a great many branches of medical science no longer bear any reasonable relationship to the expenditures involved?

And why—in spite of all our pretensions to scientific precision and clarity—does this confusion of tongues only get more confusing? So far no one has been able to provide the medical answer to these questions; perhaps, when they do, all the problems of this kind will be solved in short order. In the meantime, other approaches might be tried.

THE MYTH OF OBJECTIVITY

Historian of science Thomas S. Kuhn has compared the language of science to a box, with the practice of science thus an attempt to force all of nature to fit into this "preformed and relatively inflexible box."[20] According to Kuhn, "No part of the aim of normal science is to call forth new sorts of phenomena; indeed, those that will not fit the box are often not seen at all." Whorf advances a very similar proposition: "Segmentation of nature is an aspect of grammar—one as yet little studied by grammarians. We cut up and organize the spread and flow of events as we do, largely because, through our mother tongue, we are parties to an agreement to do so, not because nature itself is segmented in exactly that way for all to see. Languages differ not only in how they build their sentences but also in how they break down nature to secure the elements to put in those sentences."[21] Both Kuhn and Whorf argue that the very structure of language determines not only that certain phenomena and certain relationships will be *observed,* but that others will be *overlooked* as well.[22] Philosopher Wolfgang Steegmüller even maintains that the theories of "normal" scientists—in the sense that Kuhn uses the term—"are immune to all refractory experience," so that their approach to science is devoid of "even the slightest trace of the irrational."[23]

An example might make this clearer: Aristotle saw a stone swinging on the end of a rope as a case of *arrested downward motion,* whereas Galileo saw it as a *pendulum.* Both of these are instances of language-dependent observation. For Aristotle, it would have been literally unthinkable to speak of a "pendulum" or of "periodic motion," and Galileo's assertion was not based on more exact or more sophisticated methods of observation but simply on the fact that he had discarded the Aristotelian theory outright and set up a new one in its place. (In other words, he had replaced the Aristotelian language of science with a new language of his own.) Progress in medical science, as in physics and the other natural sciences, often does not result from the discovery of a brand-new fact as much as a new way of looking at a familiar set of circumstances.

26   *OLD THINGS MADE NEW*

The introduction of a new scientific language (what philosophers would call a new form of discourse, and Kuhn a *paradigm*) always has far-reaching effects, and especially so in the world of medicine. At the outset the results of whatever research has been carried out from this new vantage point are always fairly sketchy and as a rule quite irreconcilable with the established scheme of things. In contrast to this tidy matrix of theory that is regarded as well settled if not absolutely confirmed, the new language has little to offer what Kuhn calls "the promise of success." Should a scientist thus forsake this cozy theoretical edifice for the mere promise of something greater? Should he, like a grocery clerk who runs off to join the gold rush, abandon professional caution and set off into the wilderness at the first glint of paydirt?

Since the Middle Ages, at least, there have always been scientists willing to take the risk, and always in the face of spirited opposition by contemporaries who would prefer things to remain just as they are. This means that these transitional phases in the history of science are characterized by bitter power struggles that may shake an entire discipline to its foundation. One of these crises in the history of medicine took place at the end of the eighteenth century as the classical and medical doctrine of the humors was about to give way to the modern "language" of anatomical pathology and its sister disciplines. One of the leaders of the insurgent faction, a French physician named François Xavier Bichat, infuriated his conservative colleagues by the pronouncement, "With a few feverish and nervous complaints excepted, all else belongs in the realm of physical pathology."[24] Later discoveries—notably by Robert Koch in bacteriology—made it clear that Bichat was staking out a bit too much ground for himself, but he is still remembered as the founder of the science of histology.

Certainly this is not the only instance in which extravagant claims have been made for a new scientific theory. It took a great deal of laborious investigation, for example, before it was established that Newtonian mechanics could not provide a satisfactory explanation of the behavior of light. And today we still do not know whether psychoanalysis can really be of use in the treatment of certain kinds of mental illness. The limitations of a scientific theory—which necessarily implies a particular scientific language—are not always all that clear, at least until some other theory has arisen that turns out to be more effective in dealing with problems of a particular kind. And it often happens that a promising idea will be prematurely consigned to oblivion before its real merit has had a chance to become apparent—or because the appropriate "language" that would make it accessible has simply not come into being. Such ideas will often reappear much later in modern guise, in much the same way that the Cartesian doctrine of innate ideas has been resurrected in recent years by linguist Noam Chomsky.

It might be time to ask what bearing all of this might have on the problems of modern medicine. If a community of scientists sets off on a false trail, then all possibility of progress is forestalled, which is something that medical science cannot tolerate (unlike other sciences, for which progress always brings a great many fresh problems in its wake). But in medicine, stasis means that human suffering is prolonged, and in the meantime new knowledge cannot just be conjured up out of thin air. Accordingly, the medical community sometimes resorts to a rather dubious strategem: It attempts, by sheer linguistic sleight of hand, to make the concept "disease" correspond to its own current state of knowledge. This "ordinary language" definition of "illness" (formulated by Viktor von Weizsäcker) provides a good illustration of this tendency: "The essential aspect of illness is need, which manifests itself in a request for assistance. I say that someone is ill who requests my services as a doctor and whom I as a doctor recognize to be in need of them. And the determining 'category' for the assertion 'This man is ill' is—the doctor."[25]

Then what happens to those people who feel themselves to be in need but whose doctors have refused to acknowledge as "ill," as legitimately in need of their services? Weizsäcker's definition of illness seems very like a theoretical rationalization for the state of affairs described by Jores—that medical science labels large numbers of patients as hypochondriacs and leaves them to cope as best they can not only with their symptoms but with this additional social stigma as well. Such an attitude is bound to cause resentment on the part of the patient and to become a source of real conflict.

For one thing, it is axiomatic that patients are going to suffer from illnesses that medical science is incapable of diagnosing. Naturally, the treatment of an illness that cannot be diagnosed precisely is bound to be a fairly chancy business. If a doctor should happen to base a particular therapy on an inappropriate medical theory, then his treatment of the patient is likely to be inappropriate as well. The old-fashioned physician who still subscribed to the doctrine of the humors was better equipped

28   to treat a cholera patient than pioneering pathologist Bichat, with his "advanced" (but oversimplified) understanding of the nature of disease. Today the doctor who tries to bring off a miracle cure by using psychotherapy on a patient who is suffering from a liver disorder that Western medicine is still incapable of diagnosing in its early stages does not really stand much chance of success. Patients like this—if the data supplied by Jores and Schaefer can be believed—are more the rule than the exception.

THE "FLIGHT INTO THE IRRATIONAL"...

The nature of the dilemma of modern medicine should be readily apparent when we consider Steegmüller's observation that a scientist (or a doctor committed to medical science) is still behaving quite "rationally" when he clings to a theory in the face of "refractory" (and contradictory) experience. And exactly how is a scientist or a doctor expected to behave other than rationally? Does this total commitment to scientific rationality really justify the sort of intolerance that is endemic in the medical community? There is, it must be said, a kind of rationality in medical science that leads nowhere.

And if so, how can we expect to resolve this seemingly unresolvable dilemma? It is striking that practicing physician Arthur Jores reaches much the same conclusion in his critique of Western medicine as did theoretical linguist Benjamin Lee Whorf in his analysis of Western science as a whole. Both of them concluded that Western science has reached its intrinsic limitations, and no matter how much effort were to be expended in the future, very little real progress could be expected to result from it. But although Jores only hints at the existence of a fundamental error—an "oversight"—Whorf was prepared to take his analysis a step farther. He was convinced that these limitations were imposed by language itself, that it would be impossible to think scientifically in a way that would infringe or transcend the systematic "grammar" of this language. Language, "like a binding force," holds us captive. If we wish to escape from it, to discover new worlds outside the bounds of our own language, then first we must learn new languages whose structure is totally different from our own. Whorf was convinced that "users of markedly different grammars are pointed by their grammars toward different types of observations and different evaluations of externally similar acts of observation, and hence are not equivalent as observers but must arrive at somewhat different views of the world."[26]

... IS JUST A WAY OF BROADENING OUR LINGUISTIC HORIZONS

Let us now switch metaphors again and say that what we need is a different box, as Kuhn would call it, in which we can try to fit all of nature in a somewhat different way than we did before. Put that way, the task seems simple and plausible enough, and languages that have virtually nothing in common with German or English or French or Russian are not hard to come by. So we may well ask why no one so far has taken Whorf's advice.

In fact, any serious attempt to answer this question is likely to put something of a damper on our initial enthusiasm for the project. Language, in and of itself, is not the royal road to scientific progress. After all, it has taken Western science a good twenty-three hundred years since Aristotle's day to reach its present level of accomplishment, and the goal of our current project would involve a comparable undertaking, to be carried out in a considerably shorter time. A biochemist or a geophysicist or a doctor does not really have much of an incentive to learn Shawnee or Navajo in the hope of getting a fresh perspective on his subject. None of the languages that Whorf had in mind when he formulated his critique of Western science has given rise to even the most rudimentary sort of science; we might imagine (with difficulty) that mathematicians could scratch new theories from such barren ground, since these are subsequently developed on an abstract plane that is quite independent of language (set theory and group theory are two good examples of this).

THE CHINESE CONTRIBUTION

However (as anyone who has glanced at the title page of this book has probably guessed by now), we do have the thousand-year-old legacy of Far Eastern learning to help us out at this point. Chinese is, of course, completely unrelated to the Indo-European language family and, more to the point, the Chinese can also look back on an ancient scientific tradition that developed quite independently of Western science. Medicine enjoys a preeminent place among the Chinese sciences. It has had a long and distinguished history that begins somewhere around the third century B.C., and it fulfills all the criteria by which a true science can be distinguished. It is a consequential, coherent body of theory (and thus a rational science). It requires of the doctors who subscribe to its tenets that they make precise observations, and their assertions must continually be verified (which makes it an empirical science as well). Chinese doctors,

30 like their Western colleagues, arrive at a diagnosis, formulate a prognosis of the course of the illness, and base the appropriate therapy on it. Thus, just as in Western medicine, the therapeutic strategy adopted can be constantly monitored and, with the help of fresh observations, rationally corrected as well.

One way in which Chinese medicine differs from its Western counterpart is the ways in which the doctor's observations and diagnoses are expressed. Western medicine observes changes in bodily organs, analyzes blood samples, and is constantly on the lookout for "pathogens." Western medicine is based on the sciences of anatomy and histology (the study of human tissue); it is also a material science, a *somatic* (from the Greek *soma,* "body") medicine. Chinese medicine, on the other hand, is concerned with changes of state, dynamic and psychic factors, function rather than substance. The observations of Chinese doctors are based *directly* on bodily functions (and malfunctions) *without* reference to the organs, nerves, or bloodstream. Thus Chinese medicine is best suited to dealing with functional disorders—which is precisely the sort of case in which Western medicine is not always able to make conclusive observations. On the other hand, Chinese medicine can rarely be confident of success in those areas in which Western medicine is most reliable. This is not to suggest that Chinese and Western medical science should be cast in the role of competitors but rather that they seem to complement each other almost perfectly. Perhaps Chinese medicine might be of some use after all to all those patients who have exhausted the resources of academic Western medicine and are about to turn elsewhere.

EXTENDING OUR CONSCIOUSNESS

"The Western form of consciousness," C. G. Jung once wrote, "is by no means the same as *consciousness,* pure and simple. Rather it is a historically determined, geographically limited entity that only represents a fraction of humanity. The extension of our form of consciousness should not take place at the expense of other forms of consciousness; instead it should come about through the cultivation of those elements in our own psyche which are analogous to the qualities of the alien psyche—just as the East is obliged to cultivate our technology, our science and industry. The European invasion of the East was an outrage on a grand scale that has left us—*noblesse oblige*—with an obligation to gain some understanding of the East. This is perhaps more of a necessity than we may realize at the present time."[27]

When West Meets East

THE CASE OF JAMES RESTON

C. G. Jung's sage recommendation was many years ahead of his time, and since it did not inspire even his most inveterate critics to take exception to it, it was quickly forgotten. However, the kind of rapprochement with Eastern modes of thought that the great Swiss psychologist was unable to achieve was brought about some forty years later by the inflamed appendix of a columnist for *The New York Times*. James Reston was taken ill while traveling in the People's Republic of China during the summer of 1971, and at the behest of Premier Zhou Enlai, he had his appendix taken out in Beijing's Anti-Imperialist Hospital on July 17. Reston was given a local anesthetic and was fully conscious throughout the operation. Eleven of Peking's leading doctors were present, as well as an interpreter from the Foreign Ministry to relay their instructions to the patient. Acupuncture and moxibustion were used for the treatment of postoperative discomfort—"there was a noticeable relaxation of the pressure, the swelling went down within an hour, and the pain never came back."

Reston's account of his experiences as a patient in the Anti-Imperialist Hospital appeared in *The New York Times* for July 26, 1971. In response to subsequent accusations that he had staged the whole thing simply to be able to report on Chinese "needle and herbal therapy" at first hand, Reston replied crisply, "That is not only untrue, it also overestimates my imagination, my courage, and my capacity for self-sacrifice by a considerable degree."

ACUPUNCTURE REDUX

Reston's story was picked up by most of the international press, and soon the entire non-Chinese world was wondering what this curious "therapy" that involved the patient's being skewered with long steel

32   needles was all about. Acupuncture, primarily regarded until then as an irrelevant curiosity by most Westerners who were aware of it, became an overnight sensation and an obligatory topic for discussion at medical congresses and cocktail parties alike. Films and further eyewitness accounts from the People's Republic regaled us with astonishing scenes of patients on the operating table anesthetized with just a handful of needles and blithely carrying on a conversation with the surgeons as the scalpel sliced through the abdominal wall and the diseased tissue was cut away.

The notion that a defective heart valve could be corrected or a malignant tumor removed without first pumping the patient full of narcotics was truly fantastic in every sense of the word. Before any of these claims could be verified scientifically, acupuncture had become an article of faith that was hotly disputed by the skeptics and the true believers. The skeptics refused to credit what they could easily confirm with their own eyes (at least on film), whereas the true believers asserted that with acupuncture all things are possible.

The majority of doctors stood aside and assumed an attitude of skeptical detachment—which soon became difficult to maintain for many of those whose patients began to demand to know why this miracle therapy had not been made available to *them*. (Naturally, these were patients who were already on the verge of renouncing orthodox medicine for something altogether less conventional and more successful.) At weekend seminars in the cloistered atmosphere of hotels and convention centers, thousands of these doctors had their first easy lessons in plying the needle, staggered home with armloads of introductory literature, and then flew off for a quick two-week course at one of the "acupuncture centers" in Hong Kong or Taipei that had been set up at no small expense (mostly for advertising in medical journals) to instruct European and American doctors in the "thousand-year-old Oriental arts of healing."

In France, Austria, Switzerland, West Germany, and the United States, professional associations of acupuncturists sprang up on every hand and quickly developed into respectable organizations, though there was still a touch of fraternal rivalry among them. Practitioners who were not M.D.s—and who until a year or so earlier had been virtually the only ones to practice the ancient healing arts outside the Orient—were rigorously excluded from these organizations. There was nothing the M.D.s could do, however, to keep the stock of these bootleg "natural healers" from soaring during the human-potential boom of the 1970s, when theirs was to become the fastest-growing of all the healing professions. In many cases the healer's midlife career change created the sensation rather than the novelty of acupuncture itself, which wore off before too long. In West Germany, when publisher Manfred Köhnlechner opened up his "naturopathic" clinic in the fashionable Munich suburb of Grünwald, the popular press and picture magazines gave him every encouragement, and before long he had on the best-seller list a couple of books in which acupuncture was acclaimed as one of life's "instant miracles," and his naturopathic clinic waiting room was crowded with the likes of film star Senta Berger and soccer star Franz Beckenbauer.

GETTING BACK TO THE ESSENTIALS

Perhaps it was a prophetic vision of scenes like this that inspired C. G. Jung to conclude that Western man's indulgence in the mystic lore of the East was likely to prove a not entirely unmixed blessing: "Just imagine what would happen," he wrote in 1930, "if the practicing physicians, the ones who come into contact directly with suffering (and therefore receptive) humanity, had some acquaintance with Eastern systems of healing! The spirit of the East surges in through every pore, as balm for all the afflictions of Europe. It may prove to be a dangerous infection, but perhaps it might have curative powers as well. The Babylonian confusion of tongues has engendered such a sense of disorientation in the Western spirit that everyone is yearning for some simpler truth, or at least for a common fund of ideas that speak not only to the head but to the heart, that bring clarity to the contemplative mind and peace to the troubled spirit. What happened in ancient Rome is happening today as well; we are importing all sorts of exotic superstitions in the hope of finding the sovereign remedy for all of our ills."[28]

It is by no means with the intention of belittling the efforts of those Western doctors who have tried to gain some acquaintance with Chinese medicine that we observe that the way in which these American and European doctors have actually learned to practice acupuncture can at best be described as a kind of medical chinoiserie—a mass-market handicraft in the Far Eastern manner. (But in the circumstances it would be hard to imagine how things could have worked out much differently.)

BRIEF HISTORY OF CHINESE MEDICINE

The traditional Chinese art of healing began with the appearance of *The Yellow Prince's Classic of Internal Medicine*,[29] a work that is thought to

34 have been composed around the end of the third century B.C. Over the next thousand years or so, there developed a complex, fully elaborated, and highly effective system of medical science, a process that reached its peak in about the eighth century of our own era. Then, for reasons we will discuss in a later chapter, there followed a relatively abrupt period of decline beginning no earlier than the fifteenth century and that was virtually complete by the nineteenth, which was also the period in which Western medicine was first introduced into China.

Prompted by the widespread success of Western doctors in China, the Chinese elite had come to despise their own medical tradition as an antiquated jumble of pseudoscience, superstition, and "crude trafficking in herbs." Far from attempting to prevent this traditional medical science from vanishing into oblivion, the Nationalist regime was actually on the point of pronouncing an official ban on its practice, at least before a storm of protest from the provinces convinced them that the peasants would thus be left without medical care altogether. Chinese and Western medicine would be placed on an equal footing by the Communist regime. When Mao Zedong was finally in a position to carry out this promise, in 1949, academies of Chinese medicine were founded in all the major cities of China. In 1954 began the task of preparing a standard edition of all the extant literature on traditional medicine—some of which, as mentioned earlier, had been unavailable for eight hundred years or so—and in November 1958 the Central Committee of the Communist Party established the formal equality of Chinese and Western medicine. Henceforth, after a certain period of adjustment had elapsed, fully half of the personnel of all hospitals and research facilities would be free to choose between a traditional curriculum (four years of traditional study and a single year of courses in Western medicine) and a Western-style curriculum (in which the priorities were reversed).

However (as I was able to observe in many localities in China twenty years later), these sweeping political directives had been implemented to only a very modest extent. There were several reasons for this, the most obvious being the inefficiency of the Chinese administrative apparatus and the resistance of doctors trained in Western medicine, who played an influential role in the Maoist bureaucracy. Third, there were simply not enough doctors trained in traditional medicine to make up the deficit; I would suspect (as a purely intuitive and unofficial estimate) that for every candidate who was well versed in traditional medicine and who managed to pass through the mesh of the state licensing system (which had been in place then for several decades) there were fully a thousand successful candidates who had been trained exclusively along Western lines. (And since then the disproportion, if anything, has only grown greater.) Finally, there was not even a common scientific language that would enable the representatives of these two diametrically opposed approaches to medicine to communicate rationally in a clinical context. And as a technical *modus vivendi* began to be worked out between the two disciplines (as best as local conditions allowed), the overwhelming numerical imbalance in favor of Western medicine resulted in a corresponding "terminological" imbalance as well. As it turned out, the resulting compromise—which we might call a "pidgin" rather than a truly "bilingual" approach—did not really further the political goals of the project, or the scientific and methodological requirements of the disciplines involved, since, as we have already seen quite clearly, every science, every system of organized perception needs its own particular language, its own set of terminology to express its own particular way of looking at reality.

And so in the end, in spite of the Central Committee's best intentions, the directive of 1958 served only to obscure rather than cast new light on the subject of Chinese medicine. For reasons both simple and practical (and for others less simple and epistemological, and presumably unsuspected by the parties involved), this attempt to bring traditional medicine "up to date" resulted during the 1960s (and more clearly during the 1970s) in the creation of a hybrid variety of medicine that was said to be Chinese and bore a few identifiable hallmarks of Chinese medicine (in the technical and pharmacological spheres) but whose rational, theoretical foundations were no longer recognizably Chinese and eventually no longer apparent at all. The European and American doctors who arrived in the Orient with the hope of acquiring their knowledge of Chinese medicine straight from the dragon's mouth were exposed instead to a brand of "traditional" medicine in which the traditional element had been systematically distorted and almost entirely dissipated.

Since the 1970s—and the end of the Cultural Revolution in particular—a spirit of cautious revisionism has prevailed in the realm of Chinese medicine as well, and this gives us grounds for an equally cautious optimism about the future. But we will only be able to speak of a genuine, purposeful revival of traditional medicine in China when the basic epistemological problems involved are well understood by everyone engaged in the teaching and practice of Chinese medicine and, accordingly, when a program of thoroughgoing "language reform" is well under way. It will be a number of years before this can be accomplished,

36 since the rational reconstruction of the theoretical foundations of classical Chinese medicine has only just begun.

THE SITUATION IN EUROPE

A corresponding attempt at a scientific reconstruction of classical Chinese medicine had already begun in Europe—this time from the standpoint of scientific theory rather than medical practice—at about the same time European medicine had almost succeeded in exterminating traditional Chinese medicine in the land of its birth. The two great pioneers in this field were Professor Franz Hübotter of Berlin, who had been a practicing physician in China for a number of years, and historian of science Willy Hartner of Frankfurt. The outbreak of the Second World War effectively put an end to any further research along these lines, and it was not until the 1950s—thanks largely to the extraordinary impetus provided by the Chinese editors of the new standard edition of classical medical texts—that work could profitably be continued, based for the first time on a comprehensive overview of all the existing sources.

Previously a great many of the crucial texts of traditional medicine had been completely unknown—even by name or at second hand—to serious students in the West. Almost all of the technical works on acupuncture that had appeared in European languages thus far were the work of self-styled experts whose provenance was dubious or altogether obscure. This material was said to have reached the West through a variety of picturesque channels, though many of these works were simply compilations, at two or three (or even five or six) removes from the original sources. During the 1950s these authors were presented with another cache of raw material, less inauthentic but far from rigorous from a scholarly standpoint, in the form of a series of elementary textbooks on acupuncture, each produced by a collective of anonymous authors in medical schools of the People's Republic. These were issued in editions of millions of copies and were intended to provide Chinese medical students with a quick, superficial exposure to the essential principles of traditional Chinese medicine. (The original material in these textbooks consisted of extracts from the classical literature paraphrased in modern colloquial Chinese.)

Even those few translations and commentaries that were based on authentic classical sources were so badly flawed by slipshod mistranslations and oversimplifications that they served only to create fresh misunderstandings (some of which have endured to the present day) about the true nature of Chinese medicine. These translators seem to have dutifully ironed out all the linguistic idiosyncrasies of the original Chinese text that might otherwise have allowed the reader to form his own conception of the particular mode of thought that characterizes traditional Chinese science. For example, the term *wuxing* is broadly translated as "five elements," which gives no clue to its precise technical meaning, "the five transformation phases" (see page 73). And the central concept in traditional Chinese medicine, the doctrine of the function circles (which in our own technical literature we have chosen to refer to a little more succinctly as *orbisiconography*), in even the most recent works is still simply called "Chinese anatomy." This is a grotesque misnomer in its own right, which has also encouraged Western doctors to come to the conclusion that Chinese notions of anatomy remain in an exceedingly primitive state. In fact, traditional Chinese medicine has absolutely no conception of "anatomy" as such,[30] and the discipline we have called orbisiconography is in every sense the diametrical *opposite* of Western anatomy and physiology—which is to say, the systematic representation of the functional changes that take place within various regions of the body of a particular individual. As we have already mentioned, Chinese medicine consists entirely of observations of such functional relationships and correspondences, which have been elaborated into a self-contained scientific system.

In most European languages there are still a number of idiomatic expressions—so-called impersonal constructions—that evoke some occurrence or event without referring to any concrete agent of causality (I say "still" because, as a linguistic species, these idioms have generally been heading toward extinction.) In English most of the surviving expressions have to do with the weather—"It's raining," "It's snowing"—and in German you can use a portmanteau phrase like *"Es grünt"* to mean "The woods and fields and outdoor vegetation in general are turning green" without actually identifying "raindrops" or "trees and blades of grass" as the concrete source of all this activity. But apart from these occasional archaic survivals, the European languages have a regrettable tendency to be overly concrete, to introduce nonexistent "things" into what is really just a series of processes or functions. The language itself, with its insistent preference for objects over processes, implies that "vitamin deficiency" or "insufficient trace-element intake" is a "thing," like "virus," "bacteria," "localized inflammation," or "skin eruption." The difference becomes clear only when we try to observe them at first hand—all of the things in this second category can actually be seen, under the microscope, in a test tube, or simply with the naked

38   eye. In the case of so-called deficiency diseases, however, the substance in question is simply by definition not there for the scientist to observe. His perception of the "deficiency" is considerably less straightforward and can be achieved only with the help of a scientific theory that supplies him with the knowledge that a certain quantity of this vitamin or trace element is necessary to maintain a person in good health. In other words, the pathology of these deficiency disorders is based entirely on a linguistic fiction; nevertheless, medical science has been consistently successful in treating them and they no longer constitute a major public-health problem, and in this respect we should apparently consider ourselves to have been very lucky indeed.

THE RECTIFICATION OF TERMS

The phrase "rectification of terms" (*zhengming*) was first used by Confucius over twenty-four hundred years ago when he urged that every idea be made to correspond to a strictly empirical reality. "The meaning of a word," as twentieth-century philosopher Ludwig Wittgenstein observed, "is the way it is used in speech."[31] Sinologist Marcel Granet was similarly of the opinion that "it is only fitting to examine the ways in which such expressions as *yin* and *yang* were used in antiquity" in order to avoid producing a biased or unbalanced translation of a classical text.[32] Translators and commentators on classical Chinese medical texts have chosen, for the most part, to disregard this sage advice and have adopted an astonishingly inflexible and pedantic approach that not only obliterates all the subtleties and idiosyncrasies of language (a fault we have already commented on) but also imposes a misleadingly "concretized" and Westernized perspective that is fundamentally alien to the spirit of Chinese science. This in turn may encourage us as readers to read all sorts of things into the text that its ancient authors never intended, and what is more, the unparalleled completeness of traditional Chinese science is made out to be a symptom of simple ignorance. Worst of all, and presumably in the hope of evoking a reverential sigh from the reader in the presence of so much "ancient wisdom of the East," the entire text is bathed in the sort of dim, religious twilight that is thought to be suitable for "mystical" works of this kind and generally hovers just this side of total obscurity.

   And if this is the alternative, then it follows that one of the most important tasks of a scholarly enterprise of this kind is to give the reader some sense of how the language was actually used. This is a task that requires some subtlety, but the Chinese have already shown that it can be accomplished (since the difficulties faced by a Chinese editor in making these ancient texts accessible to a modern Chinese readership are not all that different, or much less formidable, than those faced by his Western counterpart). In the interim, however, even though the philological shortcomings of the existing literature on Chinese medicine have been recognized by all concerned, this has not served to clarify the terms of the public debate on the subject. Suffice it to say that both the proponents and critics of acupuncture seem to feel free to make whatever claims they suspect might be convincing, with no particular fear of contradiction, and unfortunately the general murkiness of the subject is more than sufficient to conceal the absurdity of some of the propositions advanced in this debate both from their authors and their opponents. As far as the proponents of acupuncture are concerned, the Chinese not only devised their own scientific system but anticipated much of Western medical science as well; they make the claim, for example, that the "meridian" lines that appear on acupuncture diagrams have some relationship with the organs they are named for (we will be getting back to this point in a later chapter). The critics' position is quite simply that all the claims that have been advanced in favor of acupuncture are no more than Oriental fables and fantastic travelers' tales.

A PRACTICAL DIGRESSION
The acupuncture craze of the 1970s demonstrated at least that persistent effort in a particular direction may well result in a respectable outcome, even one that is not without some significance, though the original goal of the project was by no means realized. This is not the place to embark upon a discussion of the various schools of needlework that have grown up in the West, in terms of their value either to Chinese or to Western medicine. This much at least can be said: The European and American doctors who studied acupuncture may not have gotten much closer to authentic Chinese medicine than they were when they set out. However, these doctors have since introduced a number of procedures whose efficacy, in the context of Western medicine, can no longer be doubted by any unprejudiced observer. At the same time, thousands of patients have personally experienced the soothing and healing effects of the acupuncture needles and have thus been relieved of a nagging physical ailment (or a no less burdensome regime of medication).

Critics of these various techniques of acupuncture began by simply refusing to acknowledge this record of accomplishment, and then, when the public was better informed about acupuncture and this approach was

40   no longer tenable, insisted in writing it off to "the power of suggestion," hypnotic or otherwise, and generally subjecting the claims that were made for the therapeutic and analgesic (pain-suppressing) properties of acupuncture to a much more rigorous standard of proof than they would ordinarily apply to a new medical procedure of treatment. This is merely another example of the sort of (un)scientific intolerance that according to Thomas Kuhn has chronically beset the physical sciences. This is all the more remarkable inasmuch as it would not be too costly or difficult to subject these new procedures to a definitive clinical test, perhaps where the treatment of smoking or other addictions is concerned, or anywhere else along the gamut of neurotic afflictions, from migraine to hemorrhoids. Any medical treatment that can help patients get well is "effective," and the only way to penetrate the secrets of this "ancient art of healing" is to rid oneself of preconceptions. The first of these is that traditional Chinese medicine begins and ends with acupuncture.

THE CONCEPT OF "ACUPUNCTURE"

The word itself (from the Latin *acus,* "needle") was coined at the end of the seventeenth century, after European travelers to China had observed Chinese doctors treating their patients by sticking one or more needles into their flesh. In fact there is no procedure in traditional Chinese medicine that makes use of needles *alone;* what these European observers had witnessed was part of a form of therapy called *zhenjiu,* which had been systematically developed in China over the previous fifteen hundred years or so. *Zhenjiu* means "needles and moxa"; *zhen* as a noun means "needle," and as a verb it can mean "to use a needle," "to prick with a needle," "to point out a small object with a needle," etc. *Jiu* is a word that has been used exclusively as a technical term in medicine since earliest times; it refers to the practice of burning a herb of the genus *Artemisia* (which includes wormwood and mugwort) on the surface of the patient's skin. The word *moxa* (originally borrowed from the Japanese) has been adopted in the West to describe this particular herb, and the word *moxibustion* was coined to describe the procedure itself. But for our purposes, it might be best to devise a term of our own—*acu-moxa-therapy*—that will serve as a precise equivalent to the Chinese *zhenjiu.*

Acu-moxa-therapy is sometimes referred to as "external therapy" to distinguish it from the principal form of therapy employed in Chinese medicine, the administration of prescribed drugs and other medicinal substances. Acu-moxa-therapy is said to be external because it is applied to certain impulse points (*foramina*) on the surface of the skin to stimulate particular function circles within the body—as opposed to "internal therapy," which works directly from within. As is always the case in Chinese medicine, acu-moxa-therapy is undertaken only after an exhaustive diagnosis has been made. The principles and procedures involved in diagnosis are of course quite different from what they are in the West, which is the primary difference between "acupuncture" as it is practiced in the West and acu-moxa-therapy. A Western doctor will insert his needles only after he has made a Western-style diagnosis (and presumably when diagnostic tests have proved inconclusive) or if he is following a well-worn therapeutic routine. From textbooks and his own clinical experience he has learned which impulse point (or combination of points) must be stimulated if a patient who is exhibiting certain symptoms is to be relieved of discomfort. This procedure is particularly advisable since there are no side effects of the sort that are often present when drugs are administered over a prolonged period. (Accordingly, the observation that this sort of therapy operates on a strictly prescientific basis is by no means to the discredit of acupuncture or its practitioners.)

Another hybrid variant of acu-moxa-therapy is the Chinese practice of using acupuncture needles to provide an analgesic for surgical patients (thus minimizing the risks associated with conventional anesthesia). This practice, familiar to us in the West from numerous film and photographic reports of Chinese operating theaters, has in fact become better known than acu-moxa-therapy itself. It was first developed during the 1950s by Chinese doctors, but totally outside the theoretical framework of traditional Chinese medicine (in which surgery, of course, is totally unknown), so that this "acuanalgesia," like acupuncture in the West, has simply become an auxiliary to Western medical science with an Oriental pedigree. For example, the acupuncture points in which the needles are to be inserted in this case are not chosen on the basis of an overall diagnosis of the patient (as they would be in acu-moxa-therapy) but on a strictly anatomical and topological basis, which is to say according to strictly Western criteria. In addition, the impulse point must be stimulated with an intensity that is several *thousand* times what it would be for purely therapeutic purposes if the patient is to remain effectively anesthetized during surgery.

Anesthesiologist Horst Herget, working at Justus-Liebig University in Giessen, West Germany, has developed a procedure that combines electroacupuncture with conventional anesthesia (intubation) and that was used for the first time in an open-heart operation in October 1973. This enables the chemical anesthetics that are normally used to be

42 dispensed with, for the most part, which in turn puts less of a strain on the patient. Dr. Herget's version of acuanalgesia has since been used in several thousand of the most difficult operations that have been performed in West Germany, at the German Heart Center in Munich, the Eppendorf Hospital in Hamburg, and at a number of other prestigious clinics. A great many patients who could not ordinarily have borne the risk of conventional anesthesia—perhaps because they happened to be suffering from more than one serious condition—were thus able for the very first time to undergo a critical operation in relative security. Since the effectiveness of this procedure is now a matter of public record, even the most intransigent critics of acupuncture are silent on this particular point, and this remains the least controversial of the various applications of acupuncture technique within the realm of Western medicine. Admirable as this is in theory, it does not really advance our cause at all, since this procedure bears only a very superficial relationship to the practice of Chinese medicine.

Another Western hybrid is so-called *auriculotherapy,* in which the needles are inserted exclusively into the muscle of the ear (Latin, *auris*), either for therapeutic purposes or, in more recent years, as an analgesic as well. (The effects will be felt—or not felt—in various parts of the body.) The development of auriculotherapy is frequently attributed to the Chinese, but in fact it was first described by French physician Paul Nogier in the *Deutsche Zeitschrift für Akupunktur* in 1958.[33] Nogier's findings were largely ignored in Europe, but the Chinese quickly realized that he was working along similar lines and immediately seized on Nogier's new technique and put it into practice. Later, during the acupuncture boom of the 1970s, auriculotherapy was reintroduced into Europe, along with a heady admixture of pure mythology (devised not by the Chinese but by European promoters of acupuncture, who felt that a certain element of mystery was bound to be good for business). In any case, it seems safe to say that auriculotherapy would never have enjoyed the success it has were it not for this fortuitous detour to the Orient and back and the extreme susceptibility of fashionable circles in the West to the lure of anything "Chinese."

In the interim fresh hybrids have sprung up in China and elsewhere that combine auriculotherapy with less specialized forms of acupuncture. And in addition the medical supply houses have taken to these various acupuncture techniques and have started marketing "acupuncture boxes" in which the effect of the needle is amplified by means of an electrical charge or a magnetic field. Another helpful device is the "punctoscope," which enables the doctor to find the spot where the needle is to be inserted in the first place; the latest of these developments is laseracu-puncture, in which the impulse points are directly stimulated by laser beam, thus greatly minimizing the risk of nerve damage or infection.

When we come back in a later chapter to discuss acupuncture in the context of Chinese medical theory, our discussion will be limited exclusively to acu-moxa-therapy. The extent to which these other "hybrid" imitations of Chinese medicine can successfully be integrated into a scientific medical system without a precise (or even approximate) knowledge of the original texts is still an open question. Even if these techniques cannot contribute anything to our evaluation of traditional Chinese medicine, they can themselves, on the other hand, be evaluated from the standpoint of Chinese medicine. It is primarily for this reason that this discussion of the craze for medical "chinoiserie" in the West was embarked on in the first place, because—safeguarded by the almost total inaccessibility of the Chinese classical texts—this phenomenon has given rise to so many misunderstandings and perpetuated so many enduring misconceptions.

Strengths and Limitations of Chinese Medicine

CHUNYU YI

The eminent physician Chunyu Yi lived in the province of Qi during the second century B.C. Since his interest in medicine was primarily scientific and theoretical, his bedside manner left a great deal to be desired and he became quite an unpopular figure in his native district—so much so that he was finally indicted for a heinous crime and sentenced to death. Ti Rong, the youngest of his five daughters, appealed to Emperor Wen to spare her father's life so he might atone for his great wrongdoing. The emperor asked to have Chunyu's medical records sent to the capital to give him a more objective picture of his abilities as a doctor. One of these case histories concerned an illustrious patient who was also the doctor's namesake:

> Chunyu, the field marshal of the land of Qi, was sick. I felt his pulse and said to him, "This is a case of penetrating wind, a disorder that is characterized by vomiting and diarrhea whenever one takes food or drink. You have contracted this sickness by running fast after you have badly abused your system." The field marshal replied, "I was the guest of the king, there was horse liver to eat, and I ate of it till I could eat no more. Then when I saw that the wine was being brought in, I went straight out and got on my horse and rode home. Right away I was seized with frightful diarrhea."
>
> I gave the field marshal my instructions and prescribed a draft that would restore the balance of *ardor*[34] in the certainty that he would regain his health at the end of seven days. There was another doctor named Qin Xin who was present, and as soon as I had gone out he asked of the officers of the field marshal's retinue, "What has Chunyu Yi to say about the marshal's illness?" They

answered, "He has determined that his illness is caused by penetrating wind and he believes that he can cure it." Then Qin Xin laughed and said, "He has no idea what is wrong with the marshal. According to the rule, he will die at the end of nine days." But when he did not die, his family sent for me again, and I went to see him. When questioned, he replied that my prognosis had proved to be exactly right. For seven days he had taken nothing but the healing drafts I had prescribed, and on the eighth day he was rid of his sickness. I had originally recognized the sickness by his pulse. When I examined him, his pulse fit in with the normal picture of this sickness, and the sickness developed *shun,* so that the patient did not die.[35]

(*Shun* is a technical term that literally translates "swimming with the current"—for which we have devised an equivalent term, *secundovehent.* The Chinese character that represents *shun* depicts a leaf falling into a stream, and in a medical context the word would be used to describe an event that has turned out in accordance with what is perceived as the prevailing trend or a phenomenon observable in an individual case that is following the general pattern displayed by other such phenomena—in somewhat the same way in which we might speak of an illness having "run its course.")

Clearly there are certain other aspects of Dr. Chunyu's handling of this case that require a word or two of explanation. To begin with, the technical vocabulary may seem more reminiscent of mah-jongg or a Chinese menu than serious diagnostic medicine; the term "penetrating wind" sounds especially preposterous and is by no means to be taken literally, either in the clinical or the climatic sense of the word. In reality the quaint vocabulary conceals a complete taxonomical system of qualitative conventions—that is, a series of (usually tacit) agreements that make it possible to distinguish a particular illness from others of a similar kind. It should go without saying that the way in which such a conventional system of nomenclature can be properly interpreted is by understanding the underlying conventions of the scientific community that created it. Even to the uninitiated, it should be fairly clear in this connection that Chunyu's diagnosis of "penetrating wind" does not mean that the unfortunate general was overtaken by a typhoon on his way home from the banquet. Nevertheless, Western commentators have frequently misinterpreted these normative conventions of Chinese diagnostic medicine as empirical observations (and often in an extremely facile and dilettantish fashion), and this in turn has given rise to some of the most widespread and most pernicious misunderstandings about Chinese medicine in the West (on the part of its supporters as well as its detractors). This is a subject that we will have the opportunity to go into in some detail in a later chapter; for the moment perhaps it is sufficient to point out that this system of normative conventions does exist (and that Dr. Chunyu Yi most probably knew what he was talking about).

MORE THAN FOLK MEDICINE

The example of Chunyu Yi should also help to quash another common misconception about Chinese medicine—that it is nothing more than a miscellaneous grab bag of folk cures and herbal remedies. Classical Chinese medicine is no less a full-fledged scientific discipline than its modern Western counterpart. Chunyu's own account of this case also makes it clear that some doctors, like Qin Xin, had not reached his own level of attainment and were content merely to operate "by the rules." Chunyu himself was an undistinguished student until he met his great teacher, an old man named Chenyang Qing, who advised him to destroy all the recipes for concocting drugs he had accumulated thus far and then produced his own secret collection of drug recipes to replace them. Chenyang Qing also was the first to instruct him in two of the most important medical texts, *The Yellow Prince's Classic* and the *Nanjing* ("Classic of Difficult Cases"), which was probably composed in about this period and which contains detailed instructions on arriving at a diagnosis by examining the patient's pulse.

We should bear in mind that before the invention of printing in China (which was not to occur for several centuries) the transmission of medical lore was necessarily limited and frequently passed only from father to son or from a teacher to a handful of pupils. This is part of the reason why the distribution of knowledge was quite inequitable, why an initiate like Chunyu Yi enjoyed a considerable advantage over the likes of Qin Xin. However, this is not to imply that the practice of classical Chinese medicine was any more "intuitive" or idiosyncratic, any less "scientific," than any other kind of medicine, as the following extract from Chunyu's casebook should make clear:

A king had bought a slave girl by the name of Shu in the slave market. The king esteemed her highly as a clever and virtuous young woman of many parts, and though she had always considered herself to be in good health, Chunyu was of a contrary opinion. "The servant maid is suffering from a disorder of the function circle of the spleen. She should not have to exert herself, for according to the rule when the spring comes she will cough up blood and die." When the king heard about this, he sent for the girl to come, so that he could examine her for himself. (He had not yet had the chance to sell her back again.) Still, he could see no change in her complexion, and accordingly he paid no heed to Chunyu's diagnosis. He kept this young girl in his service, but then came the spring, and one day she was walking behind the king, carrying his sword, as he went into his dressing room. When the king came out again, the girl Shu remained behind. Later the king caused her to be sent for, and they found her lying on the dressing room floor. She spat out blood and died. It happened that the sickness came upon her after she had broken out in a sweat. In the case of sicknesses that arise in this way it is the rule that the sickness will take hold of the internal organs and will be severe, even though the hair and skin still retain the glow of health.[36]

In this case Chunyu's esoteric medical lore proved to be an extremely subtle diagnostic tool, which was able to predict the onset of a serious illness long before the king—apparently a connoisseur of slave girls and presumably a well-educated layman—or the patient herself had felt the slightest hint of it. Perhaps the picturesque medical jargon is another reason why classical Chinese medicine is often regarded as a glorified compilation of folk wisdom and folk remedies. In fact, there was no great language barrier that separated the doctor from the layman (as with Latin and Greek in the West), no special terminology that was radically distinct from the ordinary vernacular. In China the educated man was distinguished from the layman by the depth, not by the breadth of his knowledge, as well as by the assiduity and intensity by which it was acquired. All Chinese education—whether of a prince or a village shopkeeper—arose from the same sources, and students who were well versed in Chinese medical science made use of essentially the same vocabulary of concepts as the rest of the population, only they were able to employ them to construct a much more comprehensive system of knowledge. (Things are no different in the West—as long as the terms in question have some meaning in the vernacular as well as the vocabulary of science.)

THE PROFESSION OF HEALING 49

But, as in the West, a doctor is expected to have other abilities besides fluency in the language of science. And in general these skills are less accessible to the common run of people—and an increase in the dispersion of medical knowledge among the general population certainly implies that doctors, as a class, have been negligent in carrying out their responsibilities (however, it does not necessarily follow that this medical knowledge is to be equated with "folk medicine"). It is true that doctors were not very highly esteemed in imperial China, partly because they constituted a commercial rather than a "professional" class, which is to say that anyone could set himself up in practice who thought he could make a living as a doctor; there were no strict standards governing medical education or admission into the profession, no supervision by the government or anyone else. "Consequently," wrote a certain Dr. A. Tartarinoff, who accompanied a Russian diplomatic mission to Peking in about 1850, "the class of doctors was always numerous in China and contained persons who were not only ignorant of medicine but innocent of even the rudiments of education and looked upon the profession solely as a means of gaining a livelihood."[37]

Not surprisingly, these doctors were treated with a measure of healthy disrespect by their patients, and it was the custom to get at least one second opinion whenever a family member fell ill. After all the consulting physicians had spoken their pieces, the family would get together and compare and discuss the proferred treatments and prescriptions before finally selecting one that seemed like it might be the most effective. This was certainly one way in which medical expertise was disseminated among the general population, though it is worth noting that (whatever the undoubted shortcomings of individual practitioners) this class of doctors still served as the collective repository of classical medical science—otherwise their patients would have created a true "folk medicine" by dispensing with their services altogether.

The sorry state of the medical profession in imperial China has also indirectly contributed its share of misconceptions and misunderstandings to the way in which Chinese medical science continues to be perceived in the West. This is simply because until the early years of our century Western observers chose to interpret Chinese medicine more or less as they found it and (especially in the absence of the elusive classical texts) to "reconstruct" Chinese medical science accordingly. Today we would not think too highly of a scholar who embarked on a comparable "reconstruction" of Western medical science solely on the basis of his

50   observations of an ordinary GP's practice or the workings of a crowded urban hospital—while ignoring all other evidence altogether (medical school curricula, medical journals and textbooks, proceedings of medical congresses, current research and scholarship, etc.). In the West at least we have certain professional standards that make it fairly likely that our observer's sample population would display at least a minimal level of competence. Traditional Chinese medical science, of course, was not protected by such safeguards, and Western observers saw nothing amiss in this technique of reconstruction, which meant that they often took the most preposterous individual lapses and vagaries to be the norm.

EVALUATING THE EFFECTIVENESS OF CHINESE MEDICINE

The first question that arises is, According to what criteria? Shall we attempt to evaluate Chinese medicine from a scientific or from a therapeutic perspective? If the answer is *therapeutic,* then the first test that any therapeutic system that differs from our own would have to pass before it could receive our unqualified endorsement would be to show that it can succeed where Western medicine has failed. In other words, this presupposes that the proving ground for Chinese medicine should be some area where all our medical science has revealed itself to be self-contradictory or has simply produced unsatisfactory results. In this connection it seems both unsporting and irrelevant to contend—as the partisans of orthodox Western medicine invariably do—that Chinese medicine should be disqualified at the outset because it is ineffective against infectious diseases. The fact is, however, that we do not need a cure for the plague, or cholera, or puerperal fever—and not just because the ones we already have are quite sufficient, but because these diseases have virtually ceased to exist in any case.

And when Chinese medicine is evaluated according to scientific criteria, then the verdict that is usually returned is no less prejudicial. Many Western doctors are of the opinion that Chinese medicine (or particular aspects of Chinese medicine, such as acupuncture and certain breathing techniques) can be acknowledged to be "scientific" only when these curious practices can be suitably explained according to the usual criteria of Western medical science. At best this is reminiscent of the attitude of an earlier generation of physicists who considered nothing to be "good science" that could not be explained in terms of Newtonian mechanics (at worst this attitude recalls the obscurantist position adopted in the days of Galileo by prominent churchmen who were anxious to stave off competition from a rival world view). We have already suggested that classical Chinese science and modern Western science embody two diametrically opposite perspectives on reality. It is in the nature of such polar opposites that they can profitably be compared but cannot successfully be invoked to *explain* each other. And in fact the current worldwide effort to provide such an explanation for Chinese medicine in terms of Western scientific concepts is necessarily bound to result not in any increase in the sum total of our knowledge in the subject but rather in the erosion and gradual annihilation of the "target" entity, which is Chinese science itself. The traditional Chinese pharmaco-poeia—which has been the object of such an investigation since the previous century, an investigation that has become particularly intensive in recent years—provides us with a telling example of this process in action. It seems that the same *materia medica* that have enjoyed an impressive record of success (in concert with Chinese diagnostic and therapeutic techniques) for several millennia, when removed from this context and reexamined in a different context (that of Western academic disputation) seem to have entirely different, sometimes unprecedented, but hardly very impressive effects (since they have hardly been tested so far) in their new scientific environment.

At this point it seems timely to recall Whorf's proposal that we should learn a totally unfamiliar language as a way of ridding ourselves of the prejudice and the preconceptions that have become attached to our usual ways of thinking and speaking. And when we not only acquire a new language but also proceed to discover a new way of observing the world, then the spectrum of possibilities is extended and we can suddenly see things that were just not there before. At the same time, new pathways of action will be opening up to us as well that will forever remain closed as long as we persist in our old, accustomed style of thinking.

EXACT SCIENCE

But if we are to explore a style of thinking that is, as Whorf says, "somehow different" from our own and remain within the realm of science, we may also have to part with our Western notions of what is and what is not "scientific." There is no cause for alarm, however, since Chinese science fulfills all the preconditions for an exact science, which is to say that it is equipped with a *clear, unambiguous vocabulary* that is organized by means of certain rules into a system that is *consistent and free from internal contradictions*. This system has specific techniques of *observation and diagnosis* at its disposal, and on the basis of these a logical,

52   coherent, and totally intelligible therapeutic system is constructed. However, Chinese science is like any other science in that it has its own standards by which it judges whether any particular method or technique that presents itself is scientifically admissible or acceptable. It would never occur to a particle physicist today to pass judgment on the current state of affairs in, say, astrophysics based solely on his knowledge of his own particular field. Instead he would simply decline to form an opinion (as most are content to do) or make some effort to read up on the subject (which in all probability would be quite unfamiliar to him) before taking a position of his own. As far as Chinese science is concerned, however, the usual sequence of first acquiring a basic knowledge of the subject and then forming an opinion seems to have been reversed; this is equally true of the partisans and critics of Chinese medicine, most of whose observations on the subject must accordingly be ruled out of court for this one very basic reason.

This is not to suggest on the other hand that Chinese medicine is simply immune from all judgment by Western science. There is in fact one reliable standard that can be applied even from afar, and that is its therapeutic success. It is worth emphasizing that patients are in a much better position to judge the validity of Chinese medicine than Western doctors are, and there are a number of reasons for this (not all of them obvious). As we have already seen, the respective strengths and weaknesses of Chinese and Western medicine overlap in a way that makes Western medicine seem best suited to coping with infectious diseases and Chinese medicine with those functional disorders and chronic illnesses in which discrete or long-term physical symptoms have not yet become apparent. Chinese medicine may seem to suffer by comparison, since these disorders are so poorly understood in the West that medical science has not yet succeeded in finding names for them, let alone diagnosing or treating them. In the past they might be tagged with such vague but grandiloquent labels as "vegetative dystonia" or "neurasthenia"; today they are merely "neurotic" or "psychosomatic" illnesses. And since these disorders remain largely unclassified or even unidentified, it is no easy task to monitor the rate of therapeutic success. For the individual patient, however, this process is considerably simplified: He feels out of sorts, senses that "something" is wrong, and is restricted in carrying out his ordinary activities. He makes repeated attempts to bring his problem to the attention of Western medical science in the person of his doctor, but without any perceptible degree of success. And then, finally, after a few sessions in a "Chinese" course of treatment, he begins to feel better—the "asymptomatic" stomach ache, chronic sleep disorder, disfiguring skin rash, or whatever it might have been is gone. And the pill bottles and all the other contents of the household medicine cabinet, formerly the principal focus of his entire existence, are suddenly quite superfluous.

Western doctors, on the other hand, view this question from a somewhat different perspective. Instead of asking, Does this treatment succeed where ours fails? they prefer a less daunting question, Can their medicine compete with the greatest achievements of Western medical science? Thus the possibility that the answer to the first question could be *yes* and the answer to the second question *no* does not even arise. But the fact remains that Chinese medicine has shown itself to be highly effective in certain areas where Western science has still not correctly identified the problems let alone found the solutions. (It is clear enough why the prospect of a whole new and undiscovered realm of sickness should be greeted less than enthusiastically by doctors in the West.) At any rate there is no reason why Western and Chinese medicine should have to compete, still less to engage in some sort of life-or-death struggle from which one will emerge victorious while the other is destroyed. Certainly a greater measure of human suffering could be relieved by both of them working together than by each working alone.

SYSTEMATIC TAXONOMY
Before we go on to discuss what Chinese medicine consists of and how these remarkable results are obtained, it may be useful to try to give a similar account of Western medicine, as succinctly and systematically as possible. First of all, Western medicine is *somatic,* which simply means that it is concerned with the human body; second, it is causal-analytic, which means that it seeks out the causes of certain phenomena, and also that it regards this particular enterprise of seeking out causes as the only scientifically valid mode of inquiry. *Somatic medicine* is based on anatomy and, as Thure von Uexküll has reminded us, is further divided into subspecialties based on particular organs or systems of the body. What medical science actually studies, then, is bones and muscles and tendons, the organs, the skin, the nerves, veins, arteries, blood, hormones, and a great deal more—all of which are substantial, material, and, in a word, *corporeal.* Thus sickness can be identified only when it brings about a detectable physical change in one of these various substances, and by the same token various disorders are attributed to the physical intervention of certain other substances—bacteria or viruses or parasites that must have invaded the body somehow, an overdose of an organic or chemical

54   toxin, poor nutrition (which is to say, for example, an intake of too much fat and too few vitamins), or the mechanical effects of some foreign object that has caused a wound.

Causal-analytic medicine implies that each of these disorders is associated with a particular cause—e.g., an infection is caused by bacteria, a hangover by alcohol consumption, a traumatic injury by a traffic accident, asphyxiation by an escape of poison gas. The point of making a diagnosis is to identify these pathological alterations and their causes and, insofar as possible, to stabilize or reverse them altogether. If this can be done before some sort of permanent and irreparable damage has been done to the patient's body, then the patient is said to be "cured." The laws of Western medicine are actually generalized assertions about which causes can be associated with which effects; e.g., "Excessive alcohol consumption causes cirrhosis of the liver." And an individual disorder is thought to have been explained adequately when such a relationship has definitely (or almost definitely) been established: "Patient suffering from liver disorder. By his own admission, patient has drunk at least four liters of wine a day for many years."

This kind of reasoning (whether or not it ultimately turns out to be correct) has two serious deficiencies, however. First, it tries to encapsulate the various, disparate agencies that cause disease in human beings in a single abstract proposition, and second, it makes the tacit and extremely dubious assumption that, at least for all practical medical purposes, everyone's liver is the same (and so are all the other tissues and organs of the body). This principle is sometimes referred to as "the homogeneity of the substrate," and it works out very neatly for doctors that a great many of the exceptions to this principle need never come to their attention—when, for example, prolonged alcohol abuse does *not* cause cirrhosis of the liver or a particular bacteria does not cause an infection. This is of no great consequence, from a medical standpoint, and in those cases where individual peculiarities manifest themselves in a general enough way, practical distinctions can be made without standing too much on principle. Adults may be treated differently from children, fat patients differently from thin patients, patients with different blood types treated differently, and so on. Still, within these fairly broad limits, the principle of homogeneity remains unchallenged.

And in those areas where this principle actually does correspond to reality (or remains therapeutically moot, as with the healthy exceptions just noted), Western medicine has undeniably been highly successful. And when this is not the case, when the causes of an illness are still largely obscure and the principle of homogeneity begins to break down, then so does Western medicine—even if a clear and unequivocal diagnosis can still be arrived at (as in the cases of diabetes, gastric ulcers, and multiple sclerosis). This is where what we have called the somatic causal-analytic method has reached the outer limits of its effectiveness, and here Western medicine can hope to do no more (at best) than suppress the symptoms, either more or less effectively.

In fact this principle of homogeneity (as far as human tissue is concerned) rests on a fairly shaky foundation, since once we have progressed beyond the subatomic level and the domain of physics and chemistry, matter gradually becomes less uniform as the complexity of its organization increases—from atoms and molecules to living cells, from the simplest one-celled organisms to individual human beings, and beyond to social, political, and cultural communities, living ecosystems, and an entire planet. It is worth noting that Western medicine has scored its greatest successes when dealing not so much with human beings as with microorganisms at the lower end of the scale—namely, viruses and bacteria. From this perspective it is perhaps a genuine stroke of luck that it is these tiny microorganisms that (in certain circumstances) can cause various illnesses in human beings and animals—illnesses that can be cured simply by killing off the microorganisms. But we also know that people are less susceptible to infection when their vital functions are in good working order, and this is something that Western medicine knows next to nothing about.

These, then, are the chief characteristics of Western medicine. Chinese medicine, on the other hand, is organized on totally different principles; it is functional (rather than somatic) and inductive and synthetic (rather than causal-analytic). It regards the human body as a system of function circles, or functional regions, which are conceived of quite independently of the particular regions of the body in which they are located. In other words, Chinese medicine is primarily concerned with functions and with movement, with the dynamic and the psychic.

Methodological Digression

A T the present moment—though it would be just as accurate to say *as* the present moment—we are experiencing a great many different stimuli of various kinds. The only way that the conscious mind can differentiate among this multiplicity of simultaneous impulses and influences is by means of their various components or characteristics— the direction that a particular impulse takes, or the "resultant" (in the very precise sense that this term is used in physics). The single distinguishing hallmark of each of these impulses is its direction, and a particular direction can be assigned to every one of the motions, functions, processes, and to each of the organic phenomena we are aware of at this moment. In fact, to assign a particular direction to such a phenomenon (or to observe a change in its direction from one moment to the next) is really the only precise objective statement that can be made about it at the time it occurs. Though it is physics, and the natural sciences in general, that are primarily concerned with such "vectors" (as any directional motion is called), which can be described relatively simply and straightforwardly in terms of the path they describe in space, the sort of vectors we encounter in the biological sciences (though no less precisely defined in and of themselves) can be *described* only in terms of qualitative, normative conventions (rather than quantitative, absolute measurements).

This should be clearer if we consider the case of a particular individual. At any given moment his or her present existence is being defined and his or her future determined by a whole complex of factors—climatic, social, and all the other "objective" conditions of daily life, as well as the current effects on his or her psychological "disposition," basic attitudes, and particular mood of the moment. Each of these factors is intimately related to what the Chinese call *zheng,* which might be rendered as "orthopathy," since it literally implies that everything is

58   proceeding "straight ahead." And by "everything" in this case is meant the totality of the body's vital functions, or more precisely the "vital signs" in which these various functions are manifested. Orthopathy is thus equivalent to the individual's capacity to maintain himself (or herself) in a balanced, harmonious, and "healthy" state of being. If this orthopathy is clearly defined (in other words, if the individual's state of health rests on a secure foundation) and the various other influences to which he or she is subject are of moderate intensity, then the individual will remain healthy. And if, on the other hand, any part of the body is deflected or diverted by disruptive internal or external influences from the overall "orthopathic" harmony of the various bodily functions, then it is said to be taking a "divergent path" (xie, or "heteropathy").

Chinese medicine, in its purely diagnostic aspect, is primarily concerned with identifying and describing this orthopathic state of an individual's vital functions, and then of course with whatever functional disturbances—"heteropathies"—may have disrupted the balance. As far as therapy is concerned, the recommended course of action may be simply to strengthen the individual's own capacity to maintain his own vital functions in an orthopathic—an integrated and harmonious—state. If this in itself is insufficient, then it may be appropriate to compensate in some way for the dysfunction, and only then, as a last resort, to attempt to suppress or eliminate the heteropathy in order to restore the patient to health.

And since what we have called inductive-synthetic science, including medicine, is concerned with both identifying and influencing the paths and directions taken by various processes—with vectors, in a word— then it must be able to track these processes as they are going on, which is simply to say that it must be able to keep track of at least two different positions (as a rule a great deal more) for each of them and *to provide a meaningful description of the relationship between them.* A great many of these will be more or less fixed at any given moment—i.e., those that involve the relationship between an individual human being and the forces of external nature and the universe, as well as those we generally denote by such terms as "character" and "heredity," and of course all the other forces that are constantly operating on the individual from within his particular geographical, social, or personal milieu. Thus the Taoist ethic envisioned the concept of "cultivating the personality" (xiushen) primarily in terms of achieving some sort of ultimate harmony between the individual and the cosmos; the Confucian ethic interpreted the same concept rather in terms of the integration of the individual into society.

In each case the assumption was that one could best pursue the project of one's development as a person by first making oneself part of the operations of some greater entity; the idea that struggling against the forces that are embodied in the world of nature or the world of men "builds character" in some way would not have been endorsed by Laozi or Confucius. Instead the complete integration of the individual personality into the external struggles and strivings of nature or of society was the classical Chinese ideal.

This is also the task of Chinese science, and Chinese medicine in particular—to construct a rational framework for one's understanding of those qualities of one's own essential being that are continually being manifested in oneself as well as those qualities that are expressed in the influences and exigencies of the world around us. (This is an approach that differs radically from the Western one, which seeks to ward off "the ills that flesh is heir to" by deliberately altering, rearranging, struggling with, or actually doing away with certain aspects of reality.) And in practice this means that Chinese medicine is concerned above all with the prevention of disease and the preservation of that harmonious balance of the individual's vital forces that we call orthopathy. Only in an exceptional case (and then only as a remedy of last resort) will the doctor attempt to restore this balance by combating the disruptive forces directly. This is fully in accordance with the maxim set forth in *The Yellow Prince's Classic:* "To cure an illness that has already [physically] manifested itself is like starting to dig a well after one is already thirsty, or forging one's weapons after the battle has already begun."

THE LIMITATIONS OF BOTH APPROACHES

As a result of their fundamentally different perspectives on reality—direct observation of current events, emphasis on functional and organic factors in the one case, and retrospective analysis of past events, emphasis on somatic and material factors in the other—Chinese and Western medicine can make their observations and then present us with two different "versions" of the same phenomenon. (Of course, the same holds true for a particular disease.) But what is really of interest here is the way in which Chinese medicine, simply by virtue of its totally different methods of observation, may be able to fill in many of the gaps in our current knowledge of medicine in the West and thus enable us to reconcile these two divergent perspectives into a single integrated and comprehensive picture of reality.

Today we are in a position to recognize the limitations of both

60   Chinese and Western medicine (though not nearly enough has been made of this opportunity thus far). The fate of millions of patients depends on how successful we are in acquainting the practitioners of Western medicine with its own inherent biases and deficiencies. Certainly the deficiencies of Chinese medicine have been apparent for some time, since they constitute the main reason for its historic decline and its problematic status in Chinese society in more recent years. Since it is primarily (and often exclusively) concerned with the current manifestations and consequences of an illness, those that can be observed in the here and now, Chinese medicine is indeed very responsive to the experience of the patient, and any sort of functional disturbance that is detectable by these methods can generally be corrected quickly, safely, and effectively. However, problems begin to arise (no matter how skillful or circumspect the physician) in those cases where the outbreak of an illness is masked for some reason (e.g., the carelessness or indifference of the patient, or another doctor's incorrect handling of the case) and the original illness is permitted to develop over a prolonged period into a massive functional disorder (which may cause an alteration in the composition of the tissues of the body and thus becomes a full-fledged somatic disorder). The Chinese themselves were quite aware of the fact that any illness that manifests itself in this way, as an alteration in the composition of the tissue, is in fact a serious, advanced, and frequently life-threatening illness. They were also aware that such illnesses required stronger, more drastic, more heroic measures than the functional disorders they were more accustomed to dealing with. And from this arose the widespread conviction that modern Western (causal-analytic) medicine is far and away more effective, since it is above all capable of coping with such serious, potentially fatal illness. And concurrently it was decided that traditional Chinese medicine, as the "weaker" and less effective of the two, was best suited to playing a strictly ancillary role, primarily as a prophylaxis, as a means of preventing a serious, life-threatening illness from breaking out in the first place.

    We are not about to dispute the essential accuracy of these two statements, but they have inspired a number of faulty conclusions and misconceptions we would certainly like to see corrected. The most pernicious of these is the notion (which we hope to have already done something to dispel) that "science" is necessarily synonymous with "causal-analytic science" (as if no other variety existed), along with its corollary, that inductive-synthetic medical science is "strictly empirical" and at best a "prescientific" form of thought. This view is not only quite untenable, it also may be a hindrance to a fuller understanding of the true nature of Chinese medicine.

CHRONIC ILLNESSES

We should not forget, however, that from the patient's point of view an illness can involve a great deal of pain and suffering without actually posing an immediate threat to life. Doctors in the West have been increasingly called upon to relieve the suffering caused by chronic illnesses (to cure them, where possible) and as well to identify and try to compensate for the sort of congenital defect that does not necessarily result in a gross physical deformity. This, as we have already pointed out, is an area where inductive-synthetic medical science (because it has learned to monitor the body's vital functions as they are actually occurring and to take note of the interrelationships among them) can deliver a prompt and unequivocal diagnosis and an accurate prognosis, and provide a form of therapy that is both effective and appropriate— while Western medical science may be unable to oblige with any of these essential services. Thus (from the Western perspective) this sort of medicine seems best suited, once again, to the task of providing early detection and prompt treatment for illnesses that (because of the diagnostic and therapeutic shortcomings of Western medicine in this respect) might otherwise reach a chronic stage, at which point even the best that Western medical science had to offer might well be of no avail.

It would be difficult to make a single sweeping statement that would accurately describe the effectiveness of Chinese medicine in treating chronic illnesses of this kind. Clearly in a case where there has been extensive damage to the internal organs, not a great deal can be done, but in general (as always) Chinese medicine holds out the possibility that the functional disorders associated with chronic illness can be exactly understood and selectively counteracted. The specificity of the diagnosis and the selectivity of the treatment not only make this approach more efficient but also manage to avoid all the side effects that cause so many problems when a symptomatic, prolonged, and largely unspecific program of drug therapy is prescribed by Western medicine. When a patient is faced with the prospect of years of unintermittent and unendurable pain, his doctor still frequently has to decide whether to provide him with superficial relief from his suffering (by means of steadily increasing doses of pain-killers) at the risk of his becoming addicted to narcotics. (The equally unpalatable alternative, of course, is simply to allow him to suffer.)

62   In Chinese medicine pain is never merely a causal symptom (which just means a sign); it is regarded as an integral component of a particular illness. Thus pain should not be treated and suppressed in isolation, since it will disappear of its own accord as soon as the particular functional agency that caused it has been identified and subsequently removed or equalized. And both these diagnostic procedures and the associated courses of treatment are well beyond the perimeter of causal-analytic science—so much so as to be no longer even recognizable for what they are apparently—and what it can accomplish in the realm of medicine. We may have much to learn from Chinese medical science over the relatively long term, but there is a more immediate lesson to be found in the history of its long decline. As with many other Chinese sciences, the limitations, the inherent biases, and the fundamental one-sidedness of Chinese medicine revealed themselves much earlier (and over a much longer period) than has been the case in the West. (The methodological rigidity of Western medicine that constitutes its greatest comparable limitation dates back only about two hundred years.) As we have seen, Chinese medicine appears to have reached its peak of development in about the year 1300, followed by a long and uninterrupted period of decadence—in spite of the fact that the central core of Chinese medical knowledge continued to be transmitted more or less intact throughout this entire time. The comparison is instructive, and it may appear that it would be just as absurd, no less unconscionable, to discard such a system outright simply because of its limitations as it would be to reject everything that is valid in the canons of Western medicine simply because its past successes have caused it to succumb to a kind of close-minded dogmatism (though this, we would like to think, is only a temporary affliction) even as it has become increasingly ineffective technically.

This brings us back to a subject we have already touched on in an earlier section, where we observed that it would not only be unscientific but also manifestly unjust to represent the deplorable state of medical practice in nineteenth-century China as somehow representative of the theoretical limitations of classical Chinese medical science. (Just as, as we have suggested earlier, it would represent the height of perversity to attempt to stake out the theoretical limitations of Western medical science on a basis of one random observation of an American "Medicaid mill" or the office of a typical European "panel doctor," where the patient encounters a pretty receptionist seated behind a dazzling white counter, hands her his so-called sickness voucher, and watches her

disappear into the unseen doctor's office. She reappears with a bottle of
worthless medicine and a signed and completed certificate that entitles
the patient to stay home from work for a week, which is just what he had
come for in the first place.)

And certainly in imperial China the discrepancy between medical
science and medical practice was a great deal more pronounced than this
(which has been a powerful, if unacknowledged factor in shaping our
prejudices and preconceptions about the effectiveness of Chinese medicine). First of all, the bulk of the population lived and died without
benefit of any medical care whatsoever; ordinary Chinese were subject to
lengthy service at compulsory forced labor (in itself a major cause of
mortality—sickness vouchers were not available). More important than
that, traditional Chinese medicine had nothing to offer in the way of
public health and hygiene (first developed along systematic lines by a
Munich doctor, Max von Pettenkofer, in the middle of the nineteenth
century) and nothing to compare with vaccination and the scientific
treatment of contagious diseases, or with surgery, for that matter; as long
as smallpox and the plague remained endemic, subtle functional disorders were of little consequence.

As we know, the situation in the West was quite different during the
nineteenth century; systematic scientific research and the practical
application of causal-analytic medical science resulted in the conquest (if
not the complete annihilation) of an entire group of epidemic diseases.
Those left unvanquished were functional disorders and chronic illnesses—which may be promoted or aggravated by stressful working
conditions, nervous tension, or psychological strain brought about by
anything from a sedentary mode of life to the unnatural disruption of
our environment to the perennial instability of our social milieu. And
these disorders, as we know by now, are the special province of
traditional Chinese medicine.

Thus we are faced with the predictable irony that in China the
demand for the services of Western medical science has been continually
on the rise, and in the West a similar demand for Chinese medicine has
been asserting itself for some time. But only the Chinese—usually made
out to be xenophobic and hostile toward foreign influences—have
adopted the appropriate social policy to resolve this paradox. They have
long since acknowledged that the kind of medical care that their
population receives should be determined by their actual medical needs
rather than by some dogmatic theoretical standard.

II

FUNDAMENTALS

Yin and Yang

I N classical Chinese thought there is no event or entity in the universe that does not have both a yin and a yang aspect. "Once *yin,* once *yang*— that is the Tao!" we are told by the *Yijing* (better known as the *I Ching*), the celebrated "Book of Changes" that formed the cornerstone of classical Chinese philosophy. A somewhat more rigorous definition is provided in Chapter Five of the first section of *The Yellow Prince's Classic,* a work known in its own right as the *Suwen,* "Book of Elementary Questions": "The Yellow Prince said this, The *yinyang* is the Tao of heaven and earth and the right rule of conduct for the ten thousand created beings, father and mother of transformation and alteration, the root and beginning of creation and annihilation, the great hall in which the constellational force is made manifest."[1]

The Tao is the way in which actions happen, the path through time and space that is taken by every event. *Yinyang,* in Western terms, means something like "equal allocation of forces," "balance of forces," "constellation of forces," as well as "polar energy," "polarized energy," and, since in Chinese thought every event is conceived of in terms of the flow of energy, simply "polarity." This much, at least, should enable us to write our own commentary on the cryptic passage from the *Yijing* quoted above: *The course of events is determined by the constellation of forces prevailing at the time,* or, alternatively, *Every event is the result of the pattern that energy assumes at that particular time.* Thus *yin* and *yang* are universal designations that can be applied to any action considered in its aspect as polar energy. On the other hand, actions can only be meaningfully evoked—can only be observed in fact—when a force (or some other form of active energy) encounters an object in space, a situation that enables some sort of change (which we call an *event*) to take place. A ray of sunlight or a meteor cannot be said to have any effect as long as they are passing uneventfully through space. And rays of

68   sunlight, which are all manifestations of the same active energy, can have many different effects, depending on the location of this interaction with an object—sunlight, for example, can supply energy for the process of photosynthesis in plants; it can cause water to evaporate, a tin roof to get warm, human skin to tan (or burn), eyelids to blink or shut tight. And clearly it is the characteristics of the "location"—the object, in other words—that define the nature of the interaction.

From the Chinese viewpoint—and this is a concept that is very deeply rooted in the Chinese consciousness—the location itself, the object, is given shape, substance, and structure in various ways by a *constructive* force, as differentiated from an active force. Thus every event is to be regarded as the interaction of an active and a constructive force, each of which has its own peculiar characteristics that determine the nature of the event. And in contrast to the sort of causal thinking that predominates in Western thought—which would contend that every event is the outcome of a cause that has already occurred at some time in the past— the Chinese would explain the same event as the instantaneous interaction of an active and a constructive force, the dynamic consummation of these two forces occurring at that very moment. The active component of every event is designated *yang* and the constructive component *yin*. And this is essentially why it is that the Chinese regard the fundamental ordering of the universe as being based on the interplay of these two groups of opposite but complementary aspects of the principle of energy. Phenomena that would be described in Western terms as "things," or objects, would instead be regarded as the consummation of a whole series of *actions,* or effects, in the past—actions that have accumulated, so to speak, in the past and are only to be sought for in the past. All material things, including the bodies of human beings, are the outcomes and the visible expressions of *quite specific* actions that have accumulated in the past, so that a landscape or a building has acquired certain *specific qualities* as the result of forces interacting over a long period *in the past*. A desert, for example, is the result of a protracted process of "desertification," and changes in the human body are the results of long-term functional disorders.

QUALITATIVE NORMATIVE CONVENTIONS

In an earlier section we used the term *normative conventions* to denote a kind of technical vocabulary that is adopted by a certain scientific community and that enables it to describe naturally occurring phenomena in their own conceptual language. More specifically, in the context of

Chinese medicine, such terms are used to enable doctors to distinguish qualitatively the diagnostically significant characteristics of those forces that act upon the human body—what we have called their directions, in other words. The famous *yin* and *yang* are extremely useful in this connection, though the original meaning of these terms was much more restricted in scope. In archaic times *yin* was used to refer to the side of a mountain that lay in shadow, *yang* to the sunlit side (hence to the northern and southern slopes of a mountain, respectively). *Yin* could also refer to the shaded bank of a river (or the northern bank), *yang* to the sunlit (or southern) bank, and, by extension, fall and winter were said to be *yin,* spring and summer were *yang.*

But terms such as *yin* and *yang* are no longer strictly empirical concepts once they have been adopted as normative conventions (the same holds true, for example, of such Western concepts as *cause* and *effect* as well). They no longer provide a description of reality as such; instead they serve as linguistic conveniences that make it easier to make empirical assertions that are both precise and unambiguous. We have already seen that *yang* no longer simply expresses the basic idea of sunlight; instead it has come to refer to the *active* component of an action or event, while *yin* is now its *constructive* counterpart, as distinguished by its material "location" in space. In addition, by a further process of extension, *yang* is also used to refer to various other transitional states, including beginning and coming into being, moving and being moved, changing, developing, and diffusing, dissolving and dispersing, determinant as well as indeterminate. *Yin* correspondingly refers to more definite or permanent states, including completion, confirmation, repose, stasis, consolidation, concentration, concreteness, and solidity (as well as contraction and extinction), and in general the state of being determinate or determined (as opposed to both determinant and undetermined).

In fact, the critical idea here seems to be that *yang,* the active principle, is also the *determining* principle, though it remains indeterminate in itself. Exactly what is meant by "indeterminate" in this instance may become clearer when we refer back to our earlier example of a ray of sunlight proceeding unhindered through empty space. It is totally *indeterminate* at this point, inasmuch as no amount of empirical investigation, however painstaking and astute, can possibly reveal what the ultimate effect of this energy will be—whether it will cause water to evaporate, for example, help a plant to grow, bounce off the moon to make it shine at night, darken a photographic plate, or merely contribute to someone's sunburn. This will become clear only when this active

70   energy encounters and interacts with constructive energy at a particular location to produce one of these effects (or perhaps some altogether different result entirely). This sunbeam, in other words, does not in itself determine what the nature of the resulting event will be, but only that it will occur.

Now perhaps we are in a somewhat better position to interpret the Yellow Prince's maxim that was quoted at the beginning of this section: The constructive principle (*yin*) and the active principle (*yang*) provide the means by which the order of the cosmos is established. All individual phenomena—"the ten thousand created beings"—are given form and substance by the interaction of these two complementary principles. Change of every kind—from transitory changes of state to deep-rooted, fundamental transformations—are brought about by the active principle, *yang,* but it is the constructive principle, *yin,* that causes everything that changes to assume a stable, concrete form (or to cease to exist altogether). Every process of renewal and decay is governed by this polarity of *yin* and *yang* and, most important of all for our immediate purposes, what the Yellow Prince refers to as the "constellational force" (that is, the force that governs and gives structure to the dynamic interaction of *events* that makes up the material universe), and all of its various manifestations can readily be observed and understood in terms of these two fundamental principles.

CORRESPONDENCES

Since Chinese scientific thought is completely dominated by these questions of dynamics and effectiveness and other operational matters, it consequently inhabits a world of emblems and symbols, of oppositions and correspondences. As we have already seen, the number of earthly and celestial objects and other phenomena that are associated with the primary principles of *yin* and *yang* may be almost limitless. "Active" phenomena that are associated with *yang* include the heavens, the sun, spring and summer, fire, and daylight, as well as anything that is regarded as masculine, warm or hot, external, light, big and strong, animated or mobile, on top, or on the left. Conversely, the list of *yin* phenomena includes the earth, the moon, fall and winter, water and rain, night, plus anything that is regarded as feminine, cool or cold, internal, dark, small and weak, still, on the bottom, or on the right. In the realm of medicine, of course, there are a number of other important correspondences and affinities. For example, *yang* is associated with, among other things, the hours between midnight and noon, anything that is on or moving toward the surface, the back, the trunk above the diaphragm, the outer function circles (passage circles), the transformation phases of wood and fire, the constellational force called *shen,* the active individual energy called *qi,* the defensive energy called *wei,* the active fluids called *nin,* the state of energy abundance called *shi* (Latin, *repletio*), as well as anything that is clear, hard, tasteless, or odd-numbered. *Yin* is associated with the hours between noon and midnight, anything that acts on or is moving toward the interior, the trunk below the diaphragm, the inner function circles (storage circles), the transformation phases of metal and water, the constructive potential *jing,* the constructive energy called *xue,* the binding energy called *ying,* the constructive fluids called *ye,* the state of energy exhaustion called *xu* (Latin, *inanitas*), plus anything that is murky or opaque, soft, savory, or even-numbered.

We will be getting back to all of this in due course, but the point to observe for the moment (apart from the fact that Chinese medicine, like its Western counterpart, is endowed with a great richness of nomenclature) is simply that a great many of these curious classifications refer to various forms of energy. It is also worth noting on the subject of *yin* and *yang* that the Chinese regarded it as self-evident that all of the phenomena we've listed could be said to have *both yin* and *yang* aspects or characteristics (that they are the sum, so to speak, of their *yin* and *yang* components). Thus we have already learned that the hours between midnight and noon are classified as *yang,* the hours from noon to midnight as *yin;* however, as Chapter Five of the *Suwen* amply illustrates, it is not quite as simple as that. "The *yin* has a *yin* inside it," we are told, "and the *yang* has a *yang* inside it in its turn. The time from sunrise to noon partakes of the yang of heaven [daylight, in other words], and this is the yang in yang. The time from noon to sunset also partakes of the *yang* of heaven, but this is the *yin* in *yang* [since the time after sunset is *yin*]. Likewise, the time from nightfall until first cockcrow [midnight] partakes of the *yin* of heaven [darkness], and this is the *yin* in *yin.* The time from first cockcrow until sunrise partakes of the yin of heaven also, but this is the *yang* in *yin.*"

The Five Transformation Phases

WE have already seen how in classical Chinese thought all events in the animate and inanimate world are conceived of as dynamic interactions that can be classified according to their polarity; the active and constructive energy principles, *yang* and *yin,* serve as the normative conventions by which this can be done. In Whorfian terms, then, *yin* and *yang* are the primary conventional criteria by means of which the continuum of reality is divided up into convenient segments—concepts—and by means of which each of these segments is assigned to a particular word as its "meaning."

Let us take a somewhat more complex example to see how this partitioning process might be carried out according to these criteria. The phrase "the hunt" should conjure up a fairly vivid mental picture to most of us (though surely without producing any general agreement as to how this concept should be logically or linguistically divided into its component parts). We begin, of course, by demarcating a *yang* and a *yin* phase for the entire process: The *yang* of the hunt begins when the stag's tracks are sighted and the chase begins; it reaches its climax when the hunter fires a shot. When the crossbow bolt or the bullet reaches its target and strikes the animal's heart, then the *yang* phase of the hunt gives way—quite rapidly, in this case—to the *yin* phase. In a matter of moments the stag will be dead, and the constructive phase, which gives rise to various new possibilities and sets the scene for new forms of activity, will begin. But before this can happen, there must be a brief transitional period in which the polarities are reversed—or in this case in which the hunter puts aside his crossbow and unsheathes his hunting knife to quarter and dress the fallen stag. (This *"yang* in *yin"* subphase is finally complete when the stag's flesh is cooked and is ready to be consumed by the hunter and his family.)

74   Clearly each phase in this orderly sequence can be further subdivided since, for example, the period during which the hunter is preparing to fire his weapon—while he draws back the crossbow and fits the bolt into the notch—qualifies as a *yin* in *yang* subphase, while the interval that begins when he pulls the trigger of the crossbow and ends when the bolt finds its target is *yang* in *yang* (conventionally referred to as the "mighty *yang*"). The moment when the bolt pierces the animal's heart begins the *yang* in *yin* subphase, and the period that begins shortly afterward, with the dead stag lying on the ground, would be called the "mighty *yin*") (*yin* in *yin,* in other words).

The fact that this partitioning of reality can be continued, in successively smaller increments, as long as patience or imagination permits may make this entire process seem both pointless and arbitrary— but of course the same thing could easily be said of the causal-analytic partitioning processes we are more accustomed to. For example, the Ems Dispatch* is generally considered to be the principal cause of the Franco-Prussian War of 1870. However, military historians have singled out entirely different events, of course, as the causes of the individual battles between the two armies, and still others as the causes of the various lesser engagements that made up these battles, and so on until we are finally left discussing the events that might have contributed to the death of an individual combatant in one of these engagements (a topic that is probably of no great interest except to those who were immediately involved at the time).

Moreover, the active and constructive principles, *yang* and *yin,* are not the only such organizational criteria in classical Chinese thought. The paired principles of *potentiality* and *actuality,* as well as those of qualitative *differentiation* as opposed to neutral, undifferentiated *uniformity,* played a scarcely less important role, particularly in the description and evaluation of cyclical events and processes, since these four principles, in various combination, give rise to the five transformation phases (Chinese, *wuxing;* Latin, *quinque transvectus*) we referred to earlier. The combination of potentiality and actuality results in a state of

---

* At the height of a diplomatic crisis in 1870, the king of Prussia met with the French ambassador at a spa called Bad Ems. The king sent his chancellor, Otto von Bismarck, a telegraphed report of their (largely conciliatory) conversations. This document—the Ems Dispatch—as substantially reworded and published by Bismarck was so provocative in its tone that the French felt compelled to declare war (which had been Bismarck's intention all along). [Tr.]

"potential activity," which the Chinese more lyrically refer to as *the transformation phase of wood*. During the hunt this phase occurs when the crossbow is taut and loaded, but the bolt has not yet been fired. (Or, to choose a more humdrum example, when the tank of a car is full and the battery is charged, the key has been inserted in the ignition, but the engine has not yet turned over.) The transformation phase of wood establishes the preconditions for a second phase, "actual activity," which the Chinese refer to as *the transformation phase of fire*. This is the time during which the crossbow bolt is in flight (or the rather lengthier period between the moment when the engine kicks over and the driver reaches his destination).

We might also have occasion to speak of a "potentially constructive" phase, in which, for example, the bolt had already struck the quarry but the stag himself was still in full flight (or the moment after the driver has stepped on the brake but before the brake shoes have engaged). This is the *transformation phase of metal*. The remaining combination, "actually constructive," is the *transformation phase of water*, and at this point the stag *is* dead (or the driver is finally *at* his destination). All of these four phases are clearly *differentiated,* however, and our second pair of new criteria are only explicitly invoked to describe those transitional interludes, "shifts of polarity," in which it is still not precisely apparent what the next phase is going to be. Such a transitional "phase shift" would include, as we mentioned earlier, the moment or two it takes the hunter to put aside his crossbow and produce his hunting knife, or perhaps the period during which the hunter is actively on the lookout for fresh tracks or a glimpse of another stag. This is what is conventionally called the *transformation phase of earth*.

The system we have briefly outlined here has frequently and incorrectly been referred to as "the doctrine of the five elements" in Western writings on Chinese science, thus perpetuating an error committed by seventeenth-century missionaries who apparently perceived a fanciful and misleading analogy between the transformation phases and the classical Greek doctrine of the four elements (earth, air, fire, and water), which had not yet entirely disappeared from European thought at that time. However, this is erroneous as a translation, or even as a comparison, in two important respects. First, the "elements" were conceived of by the Greeks and their successors partly in material, partly in functional terms (the transformation phases are defined purely

76   in functional terms). Second, to refer to a *doctrine* of five elements invokes a fundamental confusion between the purpose of an observation, the observation itself, and the means by which the observation is communicated and recorded; in other words, this is something like referring to classical Newtonian physics as "the theory of the metric system" simply because the great majority of its adherents used this particular normative convention to express their observations of reality.

(The Chinese word *xing* literally expresses the idea of "passage" or "transit," and a *xing* is always regarded as a *transitory,* or *transitional,* dynamic process whose "purpose," so to speak, is fulfilled only when it splits away or separates itself from the preceding or following process. *Transformation phase* [*transvectus*] seems to us to be the best way of expressing all these various notions without resorting to even more unwieldy circumlocution.)

At any rate, this system has an even wider application than that of describing individual processes or procedures in normative terms. The Chinese observed that these phases were likely to occur in certain fixed patterns or sequences, which naturally made them quite useful in describing dynamic or transactional systems that display a similar regularity. For example, the crossbow must be drawn before the hunter can shoot a bolt, the tank of the car must be filled up with gasoline before the driver can set off on his journey, and so forth. In other words, a phase of actual activity (fire) is generally preceded by a phase of potential activity (wood), since clearly a phase in which a great deal of energy is expended must at some point be preceded by a phase in which a suitable amount of energy is stored up.

Theoretically, there should be thirty-six such patterns or sequences of all five phases, but as far as Chinese medicine is concerned, only three of these have turned out to have great practical significance. The biological processes that take place in the human body, like all physical processes in the universe, can be regarded in terms of the interplay between an active, initiating impulse and a constructive, controlling counterforce. The active impulse (*yang*) initiates an ordered series of phases that is conventionally called *the productive sequence* (*xiangshengxu, sequentia efficiens*), in which each successive phase is said to be "engendered," or produced, by its predecessor. This sequence begins with the transformation phase of wood; wood engenders fire, then fire engenders earth, and so on, as depicted in the following diagram:

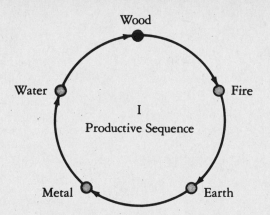

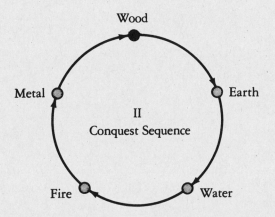

The active phases become subject to the control of their constructive counterparts in the *conquest sequence* (*xiangkexu, sequentia vincens sive cohibens*), in the course of which the transformation phase of wood "subdues" the phase of earth, earth subdues water, and so on, back to wood again.

In Chinese medicine these two sequences, and the interplay of forces they represent, are thought to form the physiological basis of all healthy, vital functions. When this play of forces is disrupted by a pathological agent of any kind, then the flow of energy becomes "congested" in some areas and is deficient in others. The result is an overlapping sequence of phase shifts in which phases with inadequate energy levels are said to be "overwhelmed" by their successors, which they themselves would normally "subdue" in the usual scheme of things. This pathological sequence of phases is called the *subjugation sequence* (*xiangwuxu, sequentia*

78   *violationis*), in which wood "subdues" metal, metal "subdues" fire, and
so on:

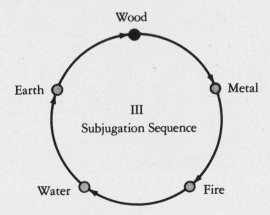

When a Chinese doctor detects such a disruption of the normal
interplay of bodily energy, then his knowledge of the various pathological
conditions that can arise from this "subjugation sequence" enables him
to make a very precise prognosis of the course the patient's illness will
take. In addition, he will already have a good idea of what medication,
or other appropriate therapy, he should prescribe to correct this
imbalance of bodily energy and thus to restore his patient to health.

III

ORBISICONOGRAPHY

The Vital Functions

BIAN QUE

The physician Bian Que, once thought to have been a contemporary of Confucius, probably lived about four centuries later, during the second century B.C. (though, as we shall see, there is still a great deal of uncertainty concerning the life and career of the historical Bian Que). As a figure of legend rather than history, Bian Que ranks with the legendary "first emperors" Shennong, "the Pharmacist Sage," "the Master of Husbandry," and Huangdi, "the Yellow Prince," among the ten celebrated "medicine kings" of antiquity. Bian Que is considered by many to have been the greatest diagnostician, and he is even said to have been able to look directly into the interiors of his patients and thus immediately to detect disorders of the function circles of the lungs, the spleen, the liver, and the kidneys. An important early medical text, the *Nanjing* ("Classic of Difficult Cases"), is traditionally ascribed to Bian Que; though probably written several centuries later, it may well bear the imprint of his own medical theories or those developed by his school. The following account of Bian Que's diagnostic prowess, which will serve as an appropriately circumstantial introduction to Chinese diagnostic medicine and the doctrine of the function circles, is not taken from the medical literature at all but from Chapter 105 of the official annals of the Han Dynasty, the *Shiji,* a work prepared by the great historian Sima Qian.

Once, Bian Que's travels brought him to the court of the land of Qi, where Duke Huan invited him to his court as an honored guest. As soon as he entered Duke Huan's hall, he announced to him, "Your Grace is sick. The sickness originates in the pores, but if it is left untreated, then it will work its way inward." "We are not sick," Duke Huan replied, and after Bian Que had gone, he announced to his retinue, "These doctors are only moved by the prospect of gain. What does it matter to

82 them if their patients are sick or well, as long as they pocket their fee?"

Five days later, however, Bian Que sought an audience with Duke Huan. "Your Grace is sick. The sickness is in the pathways. If it is not treated, I am afraid it will work its way even farther inward." Bian Que went away, and Duke Huan was troubled in his mind. When Bian Que returned five days later, he said to Duke Huan, "Your Grace is seriously ill. The sickness has taken hold in the function circles of the intestines and of the stomach. If it is not treated, I fear it will penetrate even deeper." Duke Huan gave no answer, and Bian Que went away.

But when Bian Que came for an audience given days later, he simply turned around immediately and made as if to depart as soon as he had caught sight of Duke Huan from afar. The duke sent his retainers to ask the reason for this behavior, and Bian Que answered, "When the sickness was in the pores, it could still be reached with baths and hot compresses, and when it was in the pathways, I could still have gotten at it with needles and sharp stones. When the sickness was between the function circles of the intestines and the stomach, it still could have been treated with wine and proper medicines. But now that the sickness has settled in the bones and marrow, even the Arbiter of Destiny himself [the celestial being who metes out our allotted time on earth] would be helpless against it. Now that the sickness has taken hold in the bones and marrow, there is no longer any point in consulting me." Five days later the duke was taken down with a sickness throughout his entire body. He sent one of his servants to fetch Bian Que, but the latter had long since left the district. Duke Huan died shortly thereafter.

IN THE HALL OF THE MEDICINE KINGS

"In summation: Just as the superior man knows how to interpret the preliminary signs of some occurrence in advance, so the accomplished physician is able to proceed on the basis of almost imperceptible symptoms and thus the illness is cured and the patient is spared. The great trouble with illness is that its symptoms are manifold and various. On the other hand, the great trouble with physicians is that the remedies and the ways of treating illness that they are acquainted with are few." Bian Que's biographer goes on to enumerate "the six varieties [or indications] of incurable disease," viz.:

1. arrogance and capriciousness that exceed the bounds of reason
2. insufficient regard for the integrity of one's own person, together with an excessive regard for riches and treasures

3. a propensity for improper foods and inappropriate clothing
4. disharmony between yin and yang, and the ensuing instability of the flow of active energy
5. total cachexia ["wasting," loss of muscular strength], so that medications cannot even be administered any longer
6. misplaced faith in the abilities of sorcerers, as opposed to physicians [whose treatments are based on rational principles].

"When any one of these indications is present," we are told, "then it will be difficult to do anything for the patient. The doctor should accordingly refrain from treating him altogether." Bian Que's official biographer, the historian Sima Qian, does not describe Duke Huang's case in sufficient detail to enable us to come up with a Western-style diagnosis; it seems entirely likely that modern Western medicine might have been able to do something for Duke Huang, rather than abandoning him to his fate after his illness had advanced past a certain stage. It hardly seems remarkable that modern medical science should have surpassed the sages of ancient days in this respect—but what *is* truly remarkable is that Western medicine seems to have made so little headway in the art of early diagnosis during the two millennia that have elapsed since the heyday of Bian Que.

It is also true, of course, that Bian Que's handling of this case—even with such an intransigent patient as Duke Huang—seems both unethical and incomprehensible unless we can accept the Chinese definitions of illness and health, and thus of the doctor's ethical responsibility to his patients. In the *Suwen,* an "immortal" known as the Count of Qi is quoted as saying, "The superior man does not cure an illness that has already broken out but rather one that has not yet manifested itself, just as he intervenes to quell social unrest before it has actually broken out in rebellion, before it has become manifest. To do otherwise, is this not to act too late?" We find a similar maxim in the *Nanjing:* "The good doctor treats the healthy; the bad doctor treats the sick." (Perhaps this is the basis for the popular legend that a Chinese doctor receives a fee only as long as his patients remain healthy.)

In any case, this definition of illness clearly imposes a very high standard of competence on the medical profession. A doctor is expected to be able to recognize and correctly interpret the subtlest indications of an incipient disease, long before the patient himself has felt any severe pain. This has nothing to do with sorcery or second sight. "Every illness has its own particular hallmark that appears upon the surface of the

84   body," Bian Que is supposed to have said. "The signs are not to be found
at a distance of a thousand *zi*. The decisive indications of sickness are
very numerous. One should not mistake the crooked for the straight."

These signs, the outward indications of various occurrences that take
place inside the body, are called *xiang* in Chinese, a word that can mean
both "image(s)" and "appearance(s)" (or phenomena). More specifically,
these might include a sudden outbreak of sweating, a pale face, a certain
abnormality in the appearance of the eyelids or the texture of the
fingernails, an irregularity in the feel of the pulse, a coated tongue, a
heightened sensitivity to pressure on certain areas of the skin, or a
distinctive body odor. The branch of medical science that deals with all
these phenomena (*xiang*), both in and of themselves and in relation to the
patterns displayed by such larger-scale, macrocosmic phenomena as the
weather, the cycle of the seasons, and the apparent position of the sun
and moon in the heavens, is called *zangxiang* in Chinese; since this
literally refers to the study of the "images" (or phenomena, appearances,
etc.) that are associated with the various function circles (a term that we
will be returning to shortly), we will be using the equivalent term
orbisiconography. In prescientific times, the word *zang* meant simply
"organ," a usage that has survived in modern colloquial Chinese (in the
speech of cooks, butchers, housewives, etc.). However, in a strictly
medical context it is incorrect and quite misleading to translate *zang* as
"organ" in the straightforward anatomical sense, i.e., as a collective
designation for the heart, liver, lungs, and the rest. This unfortunate
piece of terminological inexactitude has been responsible for a great deal
of confusion in the Western literature on Chinese medicine; very shortly
we shall discover for ourselves precisely wherein the difference lies.

THE "CONSTELLATION OF ENERGY"

As we have seen, Chinese medicine is primarily concerned with
dynamics, with the flow of energy, and in this respect an individual
human being is regarded as a *qi*, a particular "constellation" of energy,
rather than as a physical body that is inhabited by a soul or spirit. And
by the same token the life history of an individual is regarded as a
dynamic system, as the sum total of the interactions of a sequence of
these energy constellations. The physical sites of these dynamic events—
whether it might be the organs, the nerves, the muscles, the arteries, or
the veins—are thought to be of considerably lesser significance than the
nature of those events themselves. This is the reason why the traditional
Chinese awareness of anatomy has always seemed to Western observers

to be remarkably haphazard and sketchy; this also provides us with striking confirmation of Thomas Kuhn's suggestion that it is the nature of theory (rather than reality itself) that determines what a scientist "notices" and what he remains unaware of. Some years earlier, philosopher N. R. Hanson advanced the thesis that all scientific observations are "theory-laden" and thus that every scientist's "empirical" observations are to some extent predetermined by whatever existing body of theory he happens to subscribe to. The idea of a theoretically neutral, universally valid conclusion that would be independently verified by every scientist everywhere is simply that—an idea, a philosophical abstraction that would be sought for in vain in the real world of science.[1]

THE ORBIS

As far as Chinese medicine is concerned, the term *zang* has two distinct but concurrent meanings; first, it can refer to an actual local region of the bodily substrate, which can thus be defined (though not very precisely) in spatial and physical terms. *Zang* also refers to a particular interlocking and interdependent system of very precisely defined functions (defined in temporal and qualitative, i.e., in directional, terms). It is primarily to express this second notion that we have decided to adopt the term "function circle" (Latin, *orbis*) as its equivalent.

What distinguishes the branch of Chinese medicine we have called orbisiconography as a rational and self-sustaining science in its own right, and what distinguishes the study of these function circles from the more familiar diagnostic procedures employed in Western medicine? First, when Western doctors speak of arrested development, or exhaustion caused by stress, a sleep disorder or anxiety or nausea, abnormal hunger or thirst, then, like their ancient Chinese colleagues, they are referring to certain vital functions (and malfunctions) without actually specifying what parts of the body are involved in or affected by these particular conditions. After all, a Western doctor would also interpret a sudden outbreak of sweating (in cold weather) as a sign of illness, and Chinese doctors are not the only ones who feel their patients' pulses and ask them to stick out their tongues.

In Western medicine, however, no statement about a vital function is thought to be scientifically valid unless it is qualified by further quantitative assertions with respect to some part of the physical substrate. Western doctors are interested in assigning a cause and a local habitation to these functional disorders, and to this end X rays are taken and hormone levels tested, blood cells counted, tissue and urine samples

86   analyzed. And as far as laboratory tests are concerned, of course, it is no longer the patient who is the subject of this scrutiny, but certain suspect bits and pieces of the patient that have been removed at intervals and in various complicated ways. And if all the tests come out negative, then there is not much more that Western medicine can say about this particular patient. It is certainly possible, however, to imagine that a radio or tape recorder might have all its mechanical parts in perfect working order and still stubbornly refuse to function properly (perhaps because of some functional defect in one of its electronic components). It is just as easy to imagine that the vital processes of a human being (and thus his ability to perform to the full extent of his capacities) might be impaired in some similar way, even though the appropriate anatomical, histological, and biochemical investigations had failed to locate the source of the trouble (particularly if the real "cause" of this disorder is not to be found in the patient's blood and tissue but in his workplace or his home environment).

SYNTHESIS

By contrast, Chinese medicine is prepared to examine any functional disorder in a much broader context—that of all current micro- and macrocosmic occurrences and influences that might be of significance. In taking a patient's pulse, as many as thirty different factors or characteristics may be taken into account in determining the current state of the various function circles; there are several hundred impulse points through which the flow of energy within the body can be directly influenced by means of needles or moxa. Virtually every superficial characteristic of the body is noted and recorded—the color, shape, mobility, even the muscular tone of the blade of the tongue, the coloration, odor, moistness, slipperiness, viscosity, and stickiness of the surface of the tongue, the acuity of the sensory organs (any problem here is more likely to be regarded as an indication of a disturbance of one of the function circles rather than as a disorder in its own right), including, of course, a variety of diagnostic tests that are of great antiquity in the Western tradition as well (palpating the patient's abdomen, listening for blurred or confused speech, examining the urine and feces), and a great deal else besides.

Thus the Chinese doctor collects his basic information in just the same way as a family GP in the West—by questioning the patient. However, the information collected is by no means the final diagnosis, but only the raw data on which it is based. First, all of this diagnostic "output" must be correlated with the appropriate function circle(s), and these individual findings, like chips in a mosaic, must be assembled into a comprehensive clinical picture of this particular disorder. And, of course, the effectiveness of this procedure rests entirely on the soundness of one basic assumption—that every illness can be relied on to produce these characteristic changes in every patient, which then can be observed superficially in the rhythm of the patient's pulse, the appearance of his fingernails, or the inflections of his speech. It is also assumed that the human body will react to certain external (macrocosmic) influences in a similarly predictable way, which can provide us with certain information about the state of a patient's health. This suggests a preliminary definition of orbisiconography as a catalog of functional correspondences (between certain functional disorders and these various attendant phenomena) or as an empirically reliable system of correlating these two sets of interdependent variables.

SPEECH, SCENT, AND OTHER SENSORY DATA

It should come as no surprise that the human voice can convey a great deal of information besides the explicit content of the speaker's remarks—the signs of joy, sorrow, pain, love, hate, hope, and disappointment as well as fatigue and exhaustion and a wide variety of physical ailments. Most of us have acquired enough empirical data about our families and close associates to be able to tell when Father is having "one of his days" or when the psychological moment might be to ask the boss for a raise, but in Western medicine (apart from the very limited sense in which the subject has occupied the attention of neurologists and speech pathologists) the systematic study of the pathology of voice production has never been regarded as particularly worthwhile or important. In Chinese medicine, however, the characteristics of the patient's voice and manner of speech can provide the doctor with important information on the current state of the patient's health, since a particular abnormality may be taken as an indication that the normal flow of energy in one of the function circles is being hindered or misdirected in some way. Since the days of Bian Que, it has been recognized that a patient with a whining or "tearful" voice is actually suffering from an instability of the function circle of the lungs (*orbis pulmonalis*). The normal sequence or "tempo" of energy exchange has been disturbed, the function circle has become overloaded with energy, and its normal rhythm has been thrown off. If a patient tends to sing a great deal more than usual or insists on having music around him at all

88   times, we might take this as a sign of an accentuation of the function circle of the spleen (*orbis lienalis*), which is responsible for the distribution of energy to the various function circles and also governs the exchange of energy among them.

A patient whose speech is rambling and disconnected, who switches unexpectedly from one subject to the next, and who embarks on lengthy monologues apropos of nothing in particular is said to be suffering from exhaustion (*inanitas*) of the function circle of the heart (*orbis cardialis*). This is the function circle that coordinates all the activities of the others and that gives its distinctive and unalterable stamp to the personality of the individual. If, on the other hand, a patient merely groans or utters wordless sounds, then the function circle of the kidneys (*orbis renalis*) is affected. This is the function circle responsible for those qualities that give form and structure to the individual, both literally (the skeletal system) and figuratively (in the sense of "backbone," in other words, one's inherent disposition or character or, in Western scientific terms, the functions of the nervous system). Finally, a patient who tends to cry out loud or who is given to loud emotional outbursts is said to be suffering from a strain or an overload on the function circle of the liver (*orbis hepaticus*) in which the potential for initiating any kind of goal-oriented or purposeful activity—decisiveness, in a word—is thought to reside.

Certainly at this point a Western doctor would be tempted to ask how a predilection for groaning or singing could possibly have anything to do with the functions of the liver or the kidneys (particularly when these have very little to do with what he normally thinks of as the functions of these organs at all). First, it can hardly be emphasized too much that the function circles should not be associated with the organs they are named for in any other way, and second, a Chinese doctor would never base his diagnosis solely on the results of his examination of the patient's voice or manner of speech. He would admit quite freely that a patient's loud emotional outbursts or long, disconnected monologues were not exclusively (or even primarily) *caused* by an overload of the relevant function circle (in the same way that a Western doctor would not base his diagnosis entirely on isolated symptoms, like a fever, a headache, or a rapid pulse). Chinese doctors always regard their individual findings in the overall context of all the correlated activities of a particular function circle, and in arriving at a final diagnosis they know how to evaluate these individual data in proper perspective.

Even leaving aside the problems of malingering and deliberate deception of the doctor by the patient, it is useful to have other diagnostic data that cannot be controlled or even perceived by the patient. Thus, if a patient whose voice is observed to be abnormally shrill and whining also happens to give off a characteristic odor reminiscent of fish or raw meat, this lends credence to the doctor's initial suspicion that any further diagnostic activities should be concentrated on the function circle of the lungs. Each of the function circles is associated with a characteristic odor—pleasant and aromatic in the case of the function circle of the spleen, sharp and pungent in the case of the heart. A foul or rotten smell is associated with a disorder of the function circle of the kidneys, and a smell of urine and sour sweat, oddly enough, is associated with the function circle of the liver. All in all, there are several dozen such criteria according to which a Chinese doctor can evaluate the current state of the function circles by correlating them with, among other things, particular decades, psychic reactions, corresponding plant species, and (qualitatively) characteristic colors. The most important of these, however, was developed very early—the radial pulse diagnostic—and it is astonishing to realize how much information on the body's collective energy levels can be gathered by a skilled diagnostician simply by feeling the patient's pulse. The radial pulse is the highest tribunal, so to speak, to which every diagnosis might be submitted for final approval.

BEYOND OBSERVATION

But for this science of orbisiconography to be truly scientific, it is not enough just "not to mistake the crooked for the straight," i.e., to compile a series of accurate observations that can be correlated with particular function circles. This information must also be interpreted to provide the basis for future prognoses of the course an illness will take. Thus, like every rational science, the science of orbisiconography has at its disposal certain rules that enable it to provide a generalized and systematic description of the ongoing energy exchanges taking place within a particular "personality"—or an individual human organism, as Western medicine would have it—as part of an interconnected, dynamic structure that can be observed empirically and that exhibits certain regular patterns. Orbisiconography is concerned with describing the specific dynamic interactions associated with certain categories of illness on the one hand, and on the other hand with mapping or defining the qualitatively different forms of energy involved in the activities of the function circles. Orbisiconography is sometimes referred to as "Chinese anatomy" by Western writers, but, as we have seen, the two disciplines are only very remotely related (insofar as both concern themselves with the same

90   subject matter, the human body, but from diametrically opposite perspectives), and this seems like the sort of analogy that is more likely to cause further misunderstanding.

At any rate, this is undoubtedly one of the most impressive accomplishments of Chinese theoretical medicine—to have succeeded in correlating this vast profusion of functional phenomena (including their biological and material as well as their psychic and social aspects) with a manageable number of function circles (and to have discovered the empirical laws that these phenomena appear to obey in the process). The kind of inductive-synthetic thinking we are concerned with here has a number of distinctive characteristics, the most important among them being a reliance on direct, unmediated sense impressions and an appreciation of the cyclical nature of these phenomena. The stages of an illness (and all the other events in the life of an individual) can be systematically correlated with the sun's position in the sky (the time of day, the season of the year) and thus with all other climatic influences as well. As the *Suwen* explains, "If sickness reigns in the function circle of the liver, then it will be cured in summer. If not, it will grow worse in the fall. If the patient does not die, however, he will hold out through the winter and arise from his bed in the spring. . . . Anyone who is afflicted in the function circle of the liver will experience an alleviation of his symptoms in the morning, but they will grow worse at midday and then at midnight he will be at peace again."

The workings of the function circles are also not regarded as self-contained, homogeneous processes but instead (to use a current catchphrase) are looked at *holistically*. The function circles are thought to correspond to certain transformation phases, which, as we have seen, are associated with all manner of macrocosmic phenomena. The function circle of the liver, for example, is associated not only with spring and the early morning (hence with the east) but also with the transformation phase of wood (and thus with a great many other things besides). This also provides us with a set of rules that allow an extremely precise prognosis to be made, as well as the relevant decisions concerning the proper therapy to be administered. In and of themselves, of course, these patterns of correspondence (like much of Chinese thought in general) seem, from a Western perspective, to be totally arbitrary. It is sometimes claimed, in fact, that this sort of thinking has more in common with divination or fortune-telling than with true prediction and is thus beyond the pale of empirical science. However, as we have seen, this connection was explicitly disavowed by Bian Que, for the simple reason that he thought that patients who believed in sorcery and superstition could not be treated by more conventional means.

The question remains, however, whether these correspondence patterns and these attempts to correlate a body of empirical data with a particular function circle can be regarded as scientifically valid or meaningful. For example, why should a patient's shouting and crying out be connected with the function circle of the liver (rather than, say, the spleen)? One answer might be that this correspondence enables us to formulate a rule—that a patient who carries on and cries out in this manner is suffering from a disorder of the function circle of the liver. And why not a rule, then, that such a patient is suffering from a disorder of the function circle of the spleen? A Chinese doctor would unhesitatingly reply that the first rule is true and the second would be false, or, in other words, that the first rule has been empirically corroborated but the second has not; Chinese doctors have discovered that the first rule is a useful indicator in terms of making further diagnostic investigations. Thus it is safe to assume that for each of these correspondences there is a rule that has been verified by medical practice; conversely, when the existence of a particular correspondence is postulated in the literature that does not allow for the formulation of meaningful medical rules, then, in a medical context, at least, such a correspondence can safely be ignored. This is especially important in any attempt to separate the essential scientific core of Chinese medicine from the purely academic flourishes of the past few centuries.

THE VALUE OF THE CORRESPONDENCE PATTERNS

The science of orbisiconography allows each of the twelve function circles (there are several we have not mentioned yet) to be described, and thus distinguished unambiguously from the others, by means of some two dozen qualitative hallmarks. Together with the system of empirical rules by which the correspondences are determined (and by which the behavior of both doctor and patient become subject to scientific regulation), the science of orbisiconography is thus capable of generating an adequately differentiated picture of the functional activity of a healthy individual. Illness can be regarded as merely a departure from this normal scheme of things, and precise representations of various individual disorders can be generated in turn by the *pathology of the function circles*. However, in spite of the fact that several hundred qualitative attributes (and their corresponding rules) are involved in the practice of orbisiconography, the resulting system is by no means so complex as to

92   be incoherent or unmanageable in practice. The practical application of this body of theory is relatively simple and reliable, but on the other hand, if it is conscientiously and canonically applied, there should be no danger of oversimplification. In spite of the relative simplicity of this underlying body of rules, a Chinese doctor can arrive at a diagnosis that is sufficiently differentiated for all practical purposes—that is precise enough that two different patients would never appear to exhibit an identical pattern of functional activity. The situation is roughly analogous to the game of chess, in fact: The rules are also relatively simple, but the possible configurations of the thirty-two pieces dispersed over sixty-four different squares are virtually unlimited. Nevertheless, an experienced player may find himself in a difficult position, but never one that is incoherent or hopelessly confusing (even if, as is likely to be the case, he has never seen it before).

The Function Circles

CLASSIFICATION

Originally Chinese medical authorities distinguished eleven function circles altogether, of which five were designated as "storage circles" (*orbes horreales*) and six as "passage circles" (*orbes aulici*). The storage circles are *yin*, inasmuch as they store up constructive potential without releasing any of it. The passage circles are *yang*, and it is by means of them that liquid and solid nourishment is taken in and transformed and the active and constructive fluids (which we shall be coming to in due course) are transported throughout the body. The passage circles transmit energy but do not store it. Perhaps the best way to embark on our discussion of the function circles is simply to list them by name. The five storage circles we have already mentioned: the function circles of the liver (*gan, orbis hepaticus*), of the heart (*xin, orbis cardialis*), of the spleen (*pi, orbis lienalis*), of the lungs (*fei, orbis pulmonalis*), and of the kidneys (*shen, orbis renalis*). The six passage circles are the function circles of the gall bladder (*tan, orbis felleus*); of the small intestine (*xiaochang, orbis intestini tenuis*); of the stomach (*wei, orbis stomachi*); of the large intestine (*dachang, orbis intestini crassi*); of the bladder (*pang guang, orbis vesicalis*); and of a sixth passage circle called "the region of threefold warmth" (*sanjiao, orbis tricalorii*), which we shall refer to for convenience as the "tricalorium." (This, of course, is the only one of the function circles that is not named for a bodily organ, which should serve as a timely reminder that in the case of all of the others the connection is to be regarded as purely nominal and not as anatomical by any means.)

Even by the time that *The Yellow Prince's Classic* was being compiled, Chinese doctors had already observed a number of other functions that did not seem to fit into this schematic view of things. The result was the designation of a twelfth function circle, the *orbis pericardialis* (*xinbaoluo;* the pericardium is the membraneous sac that surrounds the heart), as

94   well as a series of six complementary "epicycles" (*paraorbes*): the function circles of the brain (paraorbis cerebri), of the spinal chord (*paraorbis medullae*), of the bones (*paraorbis ossa*), of the uterus (*paraorbis uteri*), and of the "arterial pathways" (*paraorbis sinarteriae*) (suffice it to say for the moment that these are pathways for the transmission of energy and have nothing whatsoever to do with the circulation of the blood), as well as an additional function circle of the gall bladder (*paraorbis felleus*). The *orbis pericardialis* is classified as a storage circle, and thus it serves as 'a complement to the tricalorium.

   After concentrating on theory for so long, we would like to turn now to a discussion of the wholly concrete empirical phenomena (*xiang*)—the external "images" of the function circles—that are literally the other half of the science of orbisiconography (*zangxiang*). (There are two types of phenomena that are perhaps the most important and the most characteristic of Chinese diagnostic medicine: first, the various pulse patterns associated with the function circles, and second, the mysterious "arterial pathways" mentioned earlier.[2] Since we would like to devote at least a chapter to a detailed presentation of these two topics, they will accordingly get short shrift in the following discussion of *xiang* phenomena in general.)

XIANG PHENOMENA AND THE FUNCTION CIRCLES

The former can conveniently be divided into five major groups:

1. The basic classification of the function circles as either *yang* or *yin,* the basic correlation with one of the transformation phases, and the numerous correspondences and the correlatives that are derived from these (due to the Chinese propensity for classifying everything according to those basic criteria). Bear in mind, as always, that these are qualitative (subjective) normative conventions—i.e., intended to provide a framework for clarifying certain phenomena—and not as an independent description of reality in themselves. Thus it should come as no surprise that every function circle is thought to have an "antagonist" (*zhu*) in which the normal activity of the circle is counterbalanced or reversed (in accordance with the conquest sequence of the transformation phases, as discussed in the previous chapter). There is also a qualitatively corresponding taste, an emotional correspondence (as manifested in the quality of the patient's voice) called *sheng,* an empirical designation of the quality of the

prevailing energy constellation (called *qi*), and a qualitatively characteristic color (*se*).

As far as all the various internal or environmental influences on a function circle are concerned, the basic maxim applies (with a few salient exceptions) that too much of a dose of anything can be harmful. This is a rule that was also formulated by the sixteenth-century Swiss physician Paracelsus, sometimes regarded as the father of scientific Western medicine, who wrote, "What is it that is not poison? All things are poison and nothing is not poisonous. It is the dose alone that dictates whether a thing is poison or not. As an example, every kind of food and drink may be taken in a quantity that exceeds their proper dosage, and so it is poison. The outcome makes this clear: The drugs I administer are poisonous to poison." In the latter days of Chinese medicine, however, it apparently became the custom to prescribe massive doses of drugs in accordance with a rather different maxim, which can be roughly paraphrased as "A lot helps a lot." The selection of the appropriate drug in the correct dosage (as well as an emphasis on a dietetic regime of food and drink) was much more characteristic of Chinese medicine during the classical period.

There is also a series of correspondences that are similarly derived from the five transformation phases, but these do not play a very important role in medicine. The interested reader is referred to Marcel Granet's *Chinese Thought* for further details.

2. Macrocosmic phenomena (position of the sun and moon in the sky, climatic factors, as well as the correspondences between the function circles and the times of day and the seasons) are of primary importance in ascertaining the nature of the biorhythmic activity of the total organism.

3. In the same way, the interlocking relationships between the function circles and the microcosm (the "world" within the organism) are of comparable importance. In this connection we might mention the complementary function circles (by means of which a functional linkage between a storage circle and a passage circle is sometimes created) as well as the antagonistic function circles mentioned earlier, and the parts of the body (or the associated physical activities) in which the actual functions of a particular function circle manifest themselves. The correspon-

dences between the function circles and specific pulse patterns and arterial pathways are also included in this category. The pulse patterns are exclusively of diagnostic significance, whereas the arterial pathways (as well as the impulse points they connect) are primarily important therapeutically, since they provide the theoretical basis for acu-moxa-therapy. (However, since they are especially sensitive to pain, the impulse points may also play an important diagnostic role when the normal activities of a particular function circle have been disrupted.)

4. There are a number of correspondences that can be directly evaluated as physical or sensory projections of the function circle in question, including psychic reactions (*qui; emotiones*), specific sensory organs (*guan*), and bodily orifices (*kaiqiao*) through which the workings of the function circle may be apparent.

5. Finally, each function circle is naturally characterized by a series of vital functions. In particular, each circle is permanently distinguished by a *specific* function (*zhi guan*) in the totality of all the function circles acting in concert. Many of the function circles may also take on an especially important role in maintaining and preserving the life of an individual. This is called the *fundamental* function (*ben*) of a circle, on which the life of every individual is thought to be based (and in a way that can be very precisely described). In addition, each of the storage circles stores up a particular form of physiological energy, which in turn is referred to as the *storage* function (*cang*) of the circle.

THE STORAGE CIRCLES (ORBES HORREALES)

The Commander: Function Circle of the Liver (Gan, Orbis Hepaticus)

The circle of the liver is said to be the commander of all the other function circles as well as the source of all our plans and deep reflections. The Chinese also believe that this function circle gives individual definition and visible expression to the total personality of a human being. This is because the circle of the liver serves primarily as a kind of self-replenishing reservoir of a form of constructive energy called *xue,* whose exact composition varies from one individual to the next and that is most readily apparent in tangible form as the bloodstream. The sixteenth-century physician Li Chan, who wrote a most instructive book on Chinese medicine called *Yixue Rumen,* described this situation very concisely: *"Gan* stores *xue,* for which reason it is also called 'the sea of *xue.'* If there is a superfluity of *xue,* then one always thinks that one's body is too big; if there is a deficiency, one finds one's body too small. When the eyes receive *xue,* then they can see; when the feet receive *xue,* they can walk. . . . When one lies down at night, then the *xue* flows back into *gan.* If one is indecisive in one's plans, then *gan* becomes exhausted and transmits excess heat to the other function circles. And if fluid streams uncontrollably from the nose and mouth, this means that *gan* has no more *xue* in store."

As a storage circle, the function circle of the liver is classified as *yin,* but in its dynamic aspect it is associated with the transformation phase of wood (potential activity). Since this circle serves as a kind of storage cell for the individual personality's dynamic potential for development, then any sort of disturbance in the operations of this function circle will not only affect the individual's motor abilities—the possibility of releasing the potential energy in the muscles, tendons, etc., at any given moment— but also his imagination, initiative, and even his ability to make a decision and abide by it. (This may reveal itself, as one might expect, through a diminished capacity for action and a lack of motivation, or, in quite the opposite way, in an outburst of uncontrolled, frenetic activity.) And since it is the "sea of *xue"* that is the origin of the body's motive force and ultimately controls all vital impulses, this means that the urge to take risks or to take flight, aggression or indecision, the pleasure we take in our work, and our appetite for dinner are all largely dependent on the current state of the function circle of the liver.

In this respect, Chinese doctors will naturally take care to distinguish between the symptoms of "natural" exhaustion or simple fatigue, on the one hand, and a pathological depletion of the energy of the function circle of the liver. Clearly it is perfectly normal for someone to come home in the evening after a particularly trying day or a prolonged and tedious journey and not to be able to summon up sufficient reserves of creative energy to embark on some new project. In Chinese terms this is explained as a necessary pause "for the *xue* to be replenished," or more rigorously: Since this function circle is represented by the transformation phase of wood, it prepares the way for an activity characterized by the transformation phase of fire—that is to say, in its highest stage of realization. However, assuming that everything is in good working order, the phase of fire is followed in turn by a change in polarity (conventionally represented as the transformation phase of earth), which can, as you may recall, be regarded as a neutral or transitional phase, a

98   kind of interregnum between actual and potential. If a patient shows signs of apathy and indecisiveness and of diminished physical capacity even after a good night's sleep and a normal day's activity, a Chinese doctor would probably suspect a pathological disturbance of the function circle of the liver.

The transformation phase of wood corresponds to the early morning and the spring—in other words, to the active, expansive, and thus *yang* phases of the cycles of the hours and the seasons. Consequently the function circle of the liver is designated as *yang* in *yin* (the so-called young *yin*). The hours just before sunrise and the months of February and March are the "macrocosmic" elements that correspond to the function circle of the liver; at these particular times this function circle is especially volatile and unstable, and more than usually susceptible both to disruptive influences and to therapeutic measures as well. This is useful information for the doctor, of course, and for the patient, since he has advance notice of the periods when he will be most vulnerable to disorders of this kind and can perhaps regulate his behavior accordingly. The other important "macrocosmic" influences—namely, the sort of weather that prevails in the spring and presumably in the morning as well—have a similar effect, exciting or stimulating in moderation, detrimental when they can be construed as "climatic excesses" that are likely to cause disorders of this function circle. The qualitatively corresponding taste is sour, and, once again, food and drink with a sour taste are thought to be stimulating, but only up to a certain point (where they begin to drain away the energy of the circle of the liver). A pronounced craving for sour-tasting food or drink is regarded as a diagnostic signal of a dysfunction of the liver circle.

The psychic reaction (*qing*) that corresponds to the function circle of the liver is anger, which seems to fit in very neatly with the corresponding vocal response, which is, as we have already learned, shouting and crying out. As the *Lingshu,* the second part of *The Yellow Prince's Classic,* explains it, "When the binding energy of the circle of the liver is exhausted, one feels afraid, and when it is fully replenished, then one feels angry." And it follows that it must be beneficial, in a purely physiological sense, to "let out some of your anger" occasionally, though a full-fledged apoplectic rage or a foot-stomping tantrum would naturally be regarded as too much of a good thing.

The external counterpart (*hua* or *rung;* Latin, *flos*) of the function circle of the liver may be found in the fingernails and toenails; the eyes are the corresponding sense organ (*guan*) as well as the corresponding bodily orifice (*kaiqiao*), and the flow of tears is regarded as the characteristic bodily fluid for this function circle. In practical terms, this means that the appearance and the texture (relative hardness or softness) of the nails, as well as the relative acuity of the patient's eyesight, may provide a diagnostic clue to the existence of a dysfunction in the circle of the liver. The corresponding color (green or bluish-green) of the patient's skin is not merely regarded as a metaphor, since the examining physician may detect a faint tincture of these colors (as well as a more pronounced odor of sour sweat or urine) in the course of his examination of the patient, both further indications of the same sort of dysfunction.

Finally, the circle of the liver is associated with several of the other function circles. The circle of the lungs (*orbis pulmonalis*) is its antagonist, since its physiological effects are counteracted by this circle in accordance with the conquest sequence of the transformation phases. Its complement is the function circle of the gall bladder (*orbis felleus*), and in this context the circle of the liver is described as the "inner circle" (*li; intima*) and the circle of the gall bladder as the "outer circle" (*biao; species*); these terms are only variants on the basic concepts of *yin* and *yang,* respectively.

The Prince: Function Circle of the Heart (Xin, Orbis Cardialis)

The "prince" of the circles is thought to contribute clarity of vision and direction to the total structure of the individual personality. More specifically, it produces a form of energy called *shen,* which can actively promote the characteristic structure (what we have called the "energy constellation" elsewhere) that distinguishes a particular phenomenon—in this case, which provides the internal structure and external contours of a unique individual. In the *Suwen* we are told, "Whoever gets *shen* prospers; whoever loses it declines." As a storage circle, the circle of the heart is *yin,* and since it is associated with the transformation phase of fire, it corresponds to a function that is in a fully actualized state (the hunter's arrow in midair, to refer back to our earlier example) and thus is designated *yang* in *yang* (the so-called mighty *yang*).

Thus the circle of the heart and its product or emanation, *shen,* may be regarded as the quintessence of all vital activity, of everything that takes place within the body. From a medical standpoint, the circle of the heart is responsible for the active expression of the individual personality: for all conscious behavior and for consciousness itself, for concentration and conscious coordination as well as such things as the conclusiveness of one's reasoning and the unanimity of one's thoughts—"knowing one's own mind." Functions of the sort that are represented by the transformation phase of fire and that are associated with the function circle of the heart are ultimately responsible for the fact that we can even speak of a unified, fully integrated individual personality. A disturbance of this function circle is thus accompanied by certain personality disorders—we might almost say an incipient disintegration of the personality—the initial signs of which include the inability to concentrate, forgetfulness, indifference, and apathy. If this underlying condition is left untreated, the patient may exhibit various symptoms of mental disturbance, including sleeplessness and disordered speech, epileptic seizures, and even insanity.

As with the function circle of the liver, it is quite apparent that the Chinese ascribe certain qualities to the function circle of the heart that could not possibly be more remote from the functions that this organ is generally thought to exercise in the context of Western medicine. Certainly most Western doctors would regard such problems as indecisiveness and the inability to concentrate properly as lying more in the province of psychology or psychiatry than of ordinary medicine. From the Chinese standpoint, however, the demands currently being heard in the West for a "holistic" synthesis of psyche and soma would probably seem incomprehensible, since in traditional Chinese thought the "mind-body problem" has never really been much of a cause for concern, and Chinese medicine has always dealt with the total individual, both diagnostically and therapeutically (and from a perspective that is only inadequately conveyed by the term psychosomatic). In fact, this outlook begins to seem like an indispensable prerequisite for a true medical science (and by no means merely a backdrop for some kind of prescientific speculation). The psyche is one aspect of the total function of the body and certainly one that is essential as far as our ordinary behavior is concerned. And since it is precisely this that is primarily of interest to Chinese medicine, there are in fact a great many therapeutic and diagnostic methods that we in the West would regard as *psychodiagnostic* or *psychotherapeutic* (even though, of course, these do not occupy any special niche of their own in the context of Chinese medicine), in the same way that the more "somatically oriented" methods of Chinese medicine might be designated *function-related* or (assuming that such a word existed) *function-circle-therapeutic*. This is the reason why such disparate phenomena as psychic (i.e., emotional) reactions, voice patterns, and particular forms of behavior are of such importance in reconstructing the activity of the function circles (though it is worth repeating that a Chinese doctor would never base his diagnosis solely on such "psychic" phenomena as these without employing other, more "somatic" techniques as well—e.g., the pulse diagnostic).

To get back to the function circle of the heart, however, it is interesting that the Chinese word *xin,* which literally means "heart" and is used in a more technical sense to designate this function circle, also means "consciousness" or "awareness" (the focus or the essence of the individual personality) and, in a more general sense, it conveys the idea of "midpoint" or "middle" in such compound words as *zhongxin,* "the center." In ordinary usage, *xin* is often used to mean simply "the middle" or "midsection" (i.e., of the body) and by extension "the inner man" (whatever is really essential to us, both in the sense of what we really need and what we really are), in roughly the same sense that we might say "I know it in my heart of hearts." The Western idea of the heart as the seat of the passions (at least in literary or colloquial, rather than scientific parlance) is perhaps not very far from the Chinese notion of the function circle of the heart as the active, motivating circle (again, in roughly the same way that we might use an expression like "Go where your heart leads you").

The function circle of the heart corresponds to the hours around noon (when the sun's energy is at its peak) and the summer months of June and July (as before, the period when this function circle is at its most susceptible to disorders and when therapy is likely to be most effective). A patient who has contracted such a disorder, as the *Suwen* explains, and who is not cured by late summer is likely to have a difficult time of it during the winter, but if he can hold out through the spring, "he will arise from his bed in summer." In addition, the patient "had best beware of warm clothes and hot foodstuffs." By the same token, the circle of the heart is especially susceptible to the effects of hot weather, particularly when the air is oppressively humid. And while moderate summer heat merely acts as a stimulant to the activities of this function circle, anyone with a history of instability in this respect (e.g., someone who suffers from insomnia) would be well advised to look after his health in summer and should avoid traveling in southern regions during the hotter months.

The taste sensation (*wei, sapor*) that corresponds to the function circle of the heart is bitter, which means that overindulgence in bitter-tasting food and drink will play havoc with the activities of this circle in the customary way. Unexpectedly, however, the Chinese have discovered that it is sweet-tasting food and drink, rather than bitter, that tend to drain off or deplete the energy reserves of this circle. (In general, bitter *sapores* are described as having a depressing, damping, and destructive

102 effect, whereas sweet *sapores* have a softening, moderating, harmonizing, and sustaining effect.) Pleasure is the psychic reaction that is associated with the circle of the heart, and laughter is the corresponding vocal characteristic. A superfluity of energy in this function circle will result in a display of restless, unconnected, and hectic activity, in fits of hysterical laughter, in moodiness and capriciousness, and in other forms of extreme or unusual behavior.

The primary function of the circle of the heart is to regulate the arterial pathways (*sinarteriae*) that carry *xue* (which is, you will recall, a form of constructive energy that varies in its composition from one individual to the next—a circumstance that is more succinctly described by the term "individual-specific") from its storage place in the circle of the liver; the circle of the heart also regulates the rhythm of the pulse. One unmistakable diagnostic signal of a disorder of this function circle can be observed simply by looking at the patient's face, where the corresponding color (scarlet) is more readily visible. (Certain speech disorders may also direct the doctor's attention to a dysfunction in the circle of the heart.) Sweat is the bodily fluid that corresponds to this circle; the corresponding odor is described as burning, penetrating, and pungent. The complementary "outer circle" (*species*) is the function circle of the large intestine (*orbis intestini tenuis*), and its antagonist is the circle of the kidneys (*orbis renalis*).

The Censor: Function Circle of the Spleen (Pi, Orbis Lienalis)

This function circle is the "censor" of the total organism (in the classical sense of an official who serves as the arbiter of public morality). It is also called "the sphere of criticism and reflection," the source of both creative imagination and critical insight. At the same time the circle of the spleen is also responsible (along with its complementary outer circle, the function circle of the stomach) for the digestion of the "five kinds of grain" (actually a generic term meaning "everything we eat"), and these complementary circles also serve as a storage cell for surplus energy. The circle of the spleen is associated with the transformation phase of earth, since this circle is the paradigm of the assimilation, equalization, and distribution of nourishment and the reallocation and conservation of the energy it contains—and in fact the processing of *all* the external influences and activities that an individual is required to assimilate or "digest."

So it might seem at first glance that the circle of the spleen (classified as a storage circle) has unaccountably taken it upon itself to behave like a passage circle, which processes and transmits energy without storing it. The *Lingshu* explains this task more precisely: "In the five storage circles are stored constructive potential (*jing*) and constellational force (*shen*), the polar individual-specific constructive forms of energy called *xue* and *qi,* as well as the polarized, individual-characteristic constellational forces called *hun* and *po.* Liquid and solid nourishment is assimilated and active and constructive fluids are conducted by means of the six passage circles." In the *Suwen* the circle of the spleen is specifically mentioned in connection with the passage circles (stomach, large and small intestines, bladder, and the tricalorium), which enable the process of energy accumulation and storage to take place.

The sort of equivocal, or rather executive function that is served by the circle of the spleen makes it useful as a diagnostic indicator, since if the balancing and distributive function of this circle (and its complement, the circle of the stomach) is undisturbed, this means that all of the individual's other vital functions are operating in perfect harmony. However, the exposed central position of both of these circles makes them especially vulnerable, and any sort of disturbance that is worth mentioning, which means any unbuffered shock or insult, external or internal, that can disrupt the functional equilibrium of the total individual can also put these two function circles out of action. The Chinese believe that the circle of the spleen is the primary recipient of all the external stimuli that the individual is exposed to during his entire lifetime, or, as the classical texts have it, "The function circle of the spleen is the seat of one's acquired constitutional energy [*qi ascitum*]."

As a transitional phase at the midpoint of the cycle of transformations, the transformation phase of earth is not regarded as either *yin* or *yang,* and thus, unlike the other storage circles, the circle of the spleen has no assigned polarity of its own. However, the Chinese interpret the almost unlimited adaptability of this circle as a sign of great constructive capacity, and accordingly it is classified as *yin*—in fact, as *yin* in *yin,* or the so-called mighty *yin.*

The afternoon and the late summer, "when the energy constellation of the earth is stable and has reached a peak of development," are the temporal correspondences for this circle, so that, according to the *Suwen,* any disorder afflicting this circle that is not cured during the fall will grow worse in spring and then (assuming the patient survives the spring and summer) will be cured during the following fall. The patient is advised to "beware of foodstuffs that are too rich and too warm, damp earth and damp clothing.... The sickness will go into remission at

104   sundown and grow worse again at sunrise. By midday the sickness will
be stabilized again." The propensity of the circles of the spleen and of the
stomach for bringing the activities of the other circles into harmony with
one another can be enhanced (to a certain extent) by sweet *sapores*. ("To
a certain extent" means quite a bit less than the amount of sugar and
other sweets that most Americans and Europeans are accustomed to
consuming, which has long since reached the proportions of a pathological craving or a physical dependency—and which frequently imposes a
strain on the system that can prematurely disrupt this functional
harmony of the various circles.)

The surplus energy of the circle of the spleen can be drained off by
taking food, drink, or medication that has a bitter *sapor*. Here is an
instance in which a doctor might not only fail to achieve the desired
effect but also disrupt the activities of the other circles by a slavish
application of the fundamental rule, which would lead us to expect that
a sweet-tasting substance would be the correct specific in such a case. In
fact, the circle of the spleen achieves its "highest function" (*chong,
perfectio*) in the "flesh" (*rou, caro*), the substance that gives form and
shape to the body (but that is by no means to be identified with the
muscles and tendons, which are called *jing;* see the Glossary for
additional details). In any case, an overindulgence in sweet *sapores* would
prove injurious, irritating, and ultimately destructive to this "flesh."

The Chinese have also determined on the basis of clinical experience
that the function circle of the spleen regulates the disposal of liquid
wastes. Fluid retention, increased or decreased elimination of liquid
wastes, and the inability to eliminate toxic substances by this means are
all thought to result from some disorder of the circle of the spleen
(whereas Western medicine would put the blame on various kidney
disorders, diabetes, pancreatitis, or the like). Chinese medicine diagnoses
these functional disorders not only by the edematous (puffy, swollen)
tissue that is characteristic of fluid retention but also by the "slippery"
pulse pattern (*pulsus lubricius*); these initial symptoms are followed by the
complete disruption of the process of digestion, increased expectoration
of mucus from the lungs and bronchi, irregular bowel movements,
problems with urination and with water retention in general. (In
Western medicine this particular symptom package, here regarded as a
composite portrait of the various disorders of the circle of the spleen,
would be ascribed, of course, to a great many different organs—the
intestines, the pancreas, and particularly the kidneys and bladder, but
also the lungs, the spleen itself, and the liver as well.)

"Whoever knows how to treat the function circle of the spleen," wrote
the celebrated seventeenth-century medical authority Zhang Jingyue,
"also has the power to make all the circles act in concert, since the circle
of the spleen moistens the four sides [all of the function circles of the
body] with its energy. If all the circles can partake of the binding energy
of the circle of the spleen and the latter can partake of the binding energy
of all the others, this is so because of the mutual assistance that they
render to one another." As we have seen earlier, the idea of the various
circles operating "harmoniously" and "acting in concert" is taken quite
literally in Chinese medicine, since a patient's desire to hear music or
other melodious sounds is regarded as almost *prima facie* evidence of a
disorder (particularly of some sort of strain or weakening) in the circle
of the spleen. Other evidence may include the characteristic yellow color,
or a sweetish, aromatic odor emanating from the patient's body. The
psychic reaction associated with this function circle is pensiveness or
contemplation.

In addition, the lips and the eyelids are particularly sensitive indicators
of fluid retention in the tissues and may provide the experienced
diagnostician with an important clue to the current condition of the
circle of the spleen. The mouth is the corresponding orifice for this
function circle, and its antagonist is the function circle of the liver.

The Minister: Function Circle of the Lungs (Fei, Orbis Pulmonalis)

The "minister" among the circles is responsible for the rhythmic
organization of the life of the individual and all of life's activities. The
Chinese have been aware for over two thousand years of the importance
of proper breathing (as well as the fact that the practice of an incorrect
breathing technique may bring on a wide variety of other ailments or
disorders in its wake). This is why special breathing exercises in
combination with calisthenics have been included in the therapeutic
repertory of Chinese medicine since classical times. These techniques
have also been introduced all over East Asia, largely by adherents of
Taoism. Some fifty years ago, historian Franz Hübotter described his
visit to a kind of sanitorium run by a celebrated Japanese practitioner
named Araki—"a remarkable personage with a fascinating fanatical
glint in his eye, a virtual contortionist, and a talented sculptor as well"—
in the course of which he witnessed Araki's treatment of about forty
patients of both sexes with this Taoist breath-control therapy:

By means of daily exercise sessions lasting about one hundred minutes he had brought hysterical and trembling neurasthenic patients to the point that, by the end of ten days or more, at his word of command they could slide their hands along the length of a glowing-hot iron bar that was about sixty centimeters long and a good thumb's breadth across and was fitted with a wooden handgrip (naturally, this feat was performed with great rapidity). As far as I could see, no one was ever burned.... A few of his patients had progressed so far that they could actually stand upon and walk barefoot along the blades of long, sharp Japanese swords that were set side by side in a special wooden rack devised for this purpose (with the cutting edges facing upward). Araki presented me with one of these swords as a memento of the occasion. I have no plausible explanation for this, and Araki maintained for his part that the participants were actually suffused with the Tao of Heaven and, by virtue of having performed the appropriate breathing exercises beforehand, were thus protected from any injury.[3]

Certainly these picturesque activities are by no means prescribed as standard treatment for nervous complaints in orthodox Chinese medical practice, but there is one interesting connection between Araki's Taoist showmanship and Chinese medical theory. According to the *Suwen,* the circle of the lungs controls that function of the skin that "encloses the flesh of the muscles and tendons and wards off all pernicious influences." In dynamic terms, the circle of the lungs is the origin of a form of constellational energy that is organized by means of the rhythm of respiration; the circle acts as a storage cell for "individual-characteristic active binding forces."

Today, as visitors to China and devoted viewers of television documentaries are well aware, it is no longer necessary to seek out the lair of a Taoist ascetic like Araki to observe this ancient doctrine of rhythmic breathing being put into practice in a contemporary context. The sight of large groups of Chinese of assorted ages dutifully practicing these exercises in all weathers and at any hour of the day in parks and public squares is one of the most striking images we have of daily life in the People's Republic. A more demanding set of exercises are employed in the treatment of certain illnesses. These are called *qiqong,* "*qi* exercises," or, in other words, "active energy exercises," and an analytically inclined observer might be able to distinguish separate elements of meditation, breath control, and gymnastics. And, of course, the most famous variety of *qi* exercise is *taijiquan* (literally, "fistfighting of the topmost pinnacle," more frequently encountered as *tai ch'i chuan*), which was perfected in the nineteenth century in China and which has twice been successfully transplanted to the West, first in the form of a hybrid universally known as "shadowboxing" and more recently as a system of martial-arts exercises in its own right.

The basic purpose of all these activities is to impose a disciplined, rhythmic pattern on one's body movements and thus indirectly (and involuntarily) to influence the rate and quality of respiration (though it is worth bearing in mind that both the purpose and the benefits of these exercises, particularly the more challenging ones, are not so narrowly circumscribed). To begin with, a great many of the rhythms or regulatory functions that Chinese medicine attributes to the circle of the lungs have nothing to do with respiration (as conceived of by Western medicine). Prominent among these are those physiological rhythms that have their sources outside the individual—i.e., the cycles of the days and of the seasons, or what we might call the rhythms of daily life. Irregularities in the latter, especially in one's sleeping cycle (such as might be experienced by workers changing shifts, for example), may if prolonged over weeks or months have just as detrimental an effect on the functioning of the circle of the lungs as improper breath control. Such dysfunctions can, with the help of a therapist, be transferred from one's unconscious to one's conscious control by means of a technique that has lately come to be called "autonomic learning" in the West; then they can be corrected through exercise and instruction, and finally transferred back to one's involuntary control once the function has been successfully "debugged."

The physiological effects of poor posture and other bad kinesthetic habits have also received a great deal of attention in the West in recent decades, but in Chinese medicine these are primarily regarded as harmful because they increase the susceptibility of the function circle of the lungs to colds, "chills," the flu, and a number of other illnesses as well. It is also regarded as important to regulate the rhythm of one's daily activities in accordance with the seasons; in summer one should lead an active life and need not worry too much about sleep, but in winter one should restrict one's activities somewhat and get more rest. (This is simply a reflection of the fact that the days are shorter in winter, and the requirements of the function circle of the lungs are thought to vary accordingly.) Once again, we may occasionally hear in the West of the effects of "biorhythms" or "circadian rhythms" on human physiology, but for the most part in societies where the prevailing conception of physiology is purely mechanistic, such elementary rules as these are much more honored in the breach than in the observance.

This question of the rhythmic harmony of the body (or the lack thereof) is addressed in *The Yellow Prince's Classic* in an interesting fashion. At one point the Yellow Prince asks of his mentor, the Count of Qi: "I have heard that men in ancient times lived to the age of one hundred, and without any diminution of their physical capacities. But in our times men's powers begin to decline when they are scarcely half that age. Is the reason for this to be found simply in the difference in the times and the generations, or has there been a decline in the capacities of the individual man?"

"The men of ancient times," the count replies, "were well acquainted with the Tao. They oriented themselves correctly with respect to *yin* and *yang* and sought harmony through the useful arts and the mastery of numbers. They ate and drank in moderation, and in the conduct of their lives they followed an unvarying rule. They shunned vain strivings and heedless exertions, so that like demigods, they were able to retain their bodily forms throughout the span of years that is ordained by Heaven and only forsook this earthly existence after they had reached a hundred.... What prevents our contemporaries from living as long as the ancients is this striving after conscious pleasure while neglecting to familiarize themselves with the laws of nature and to submit to them. This means that one's constitutional energy potential is continually being overtaxed, binding energy is dissipated, and orthopathy is progressively diminished and destroyed."

In the cycle of the transformation phases the circle of the lungs is associated with the transformation phase of metal (constructive potential) and is classified as "young *yin*" (*yin* in *yang*) or even occasionally as "young *yin* in *yang*." This circle is associated with sharp-tasting substances; the corresponding psychic reaction is sorrow, and the accompanying vocal characteristic is weeping. This circle is particularly sensitive (both to functional disorders and to therapeutic influences as well) during the late afternoon and early evening (and during the fall). The *Suwen* explains that disorders of this function circle are likely to improve during the winter, then to grow worse again during the summer, and finally, if the patient survives the summer, to stabilize during the late summer. "The patient will arise from his bed in the fall. He should beware of cold food and cold drinks, and clothing that lets the cold in." Similarly, according to the *Suwen,* a disorder of this circle can be expected to go into remission during

the afternoon, then to grow worse again the following midday. "At
midnight the patient will find rest."

As implied earlier, in our brief commentary on Araki and his patients, the circle of the lungs finds its "highest function" in the skin, which, as in Western medicine, is regarded as the individual's first line of defense against noxious external influences. It is also regarded as the domain of the body's defensive energy (*weiqi*), which exercises all of its functions through the skin. Consequently, if the functions of the circle of the lungs are imperiled, this can most easily be confirmed diagnostically by observing the skin—whether it is especially reddened or pallid, moist or dry to the touch, whether or not there is gooseflesh ("out of season," as it were) or an abnormal secretion of sweat (or an abnormal *absence* of sweating). All of these will enable the doctor to draw certain inferences concerning the current state of the circle of the lungs.

The color that is associated with this circle is white; the corresponding bodily fluid is nasal mucus, and the nose is both the corresponding sensory organ and the corresponding bodily orifice. The corresponding odor is generally likened to that of raw meat or fish. The circle of the heart is its antagonist, the circle of the large intestine its complementary outer circle.

Mighty Official: Function Circle of the Kidneys (Shen, Orbis Renalis)

The function circle of the kidneys is sometimes referred to as the "mighty official" among the circles (literally, "the authority of exponential power," *zuoqiang zhi guan*), since it is the storehouse of the individual's inherent power and his natural gifts. It is here as well that everything acquired by rational study throughout the course of the individual's lifetime is preserved, so that it also forms the basis of long-term memory. The circle of the kidneys is associated with the transformation phase of water (the constructive principle at the highest level of actualization, as represented in our earlier concrete examples by the quarry's lying dead at the hunter's feet or the driver's having reached his destination). The circle of the kidneys is regarded as the source of the body's resistance and endurance, of physical, emotional, and spiritual tenacity. The makeup of this function circle largely determines whether a man or a woman can withstand physical exertion and mental anguish, nervous strain and stressful circumstances, whether he or she can endure extreme cold or extreme heat. And by the same token, anyone who is easily tired out, easily confused or upset, is likely to be suspected of some deficiency in this area, and a prolonged depletion of the energy of this

110   function circle is thought to result in the disintegration of the personality, total disorientation, and insanity. The reason for this is that all those functions that Western medicine ascribes to the brain and the rest of the nervous system are classified in Chinese medicine as functions of the circle of the kidneys.

In fact, the circle of the kidneys is regarded as the storehouse of all those qualities and abilities we may transmit to our posterity through those mechanisms of procreation and heredity. Accordingly, one of the most vital functions of this circle is sexual potency (or fertility, as the case might be), and a deficiency or disturbance in this function circle almost always implies some sort of sexual dysfunction. And in accordance with the axiom that anything that corresponds to a particular function circle is beneficial in moderate amounts and harmful when taken to excess, a life of unrestrained sexual debauchery will also result in an impairment of all the other functions of the circle of the kidneys.

It is essential here not to lose sight of one all-important point, namely that the Chinese do not, of course, go so far as to maintain that the kidneys are the "seat of memory" (or of procreation, for that matter) in the sense that such a phrase might be used in the context of Western anatomy or physiology. Nor do they maintain that these are in any sense "functions" of these organs—as both critics and superficial adepts of Chinese medicine have frequently asserted. Instead, Chinese medicine has assembled all the dynamic aspects of the constructive principle in its highest stage of actualization or completion—what might be thought of as the deepest, most ancient strata in the physical makeup and personality of every individual—into a single function circle that has been given the name *shen,* the circle of the kidneys. However, as far as Chinese medicine is concerned, the function circle has very little to do (virtually nothing in this case) with the organ it is named for; to maintain otherwise would be tantamount to asserting that the Chinese believe that the huntsman's arrow actually bursts into flame the moment it leaves his bowstring (because the activity of "hunting" has now entered a phase that is designated the "transformation phase of fire").

Practitioners of traditional Chinese medicine claim to have amassed considerable diagnostic and therapeutic evidence for this contention that the various aspects of the individual's capacity for resistance or endurance, as well as the aggregate of his or her inherited and acquired capacities, can be grouped together in a single function circle. This presents a striking parallel to the viewpoint adopted in recent years by the Western science of embryology, which has also discovered certain developmental connections (both phylogenetic and ontogenetic—i.e., concerned with the developmental history of both the individual and the species) between certain organs and systemic functions that could not be adequately explained on the basis of our current understanding of anatomy or physiology. We need think only of the developmental connection between the gonads and the embryological structure that develops into the kidneys, for example, or of the characteristics these have in common with the embryological nervous system. The nervous system, with its extremely slow metabolic rate, and the bones and teeth, for which the same holds true, can be grouped together as the oldest stratum of ontogenetic and phylogenetic development; this in itself should perhaps not be regarded as "confirmation" of Chinese medical theory, but it suggests that this complex system of functions and correspondences may not be quite as arbitrary as it sometimes seems to Western eyes.

The function circle of the kidneys is associated with the transformation phase of water, which refers, we hasten to add, exclusively to the individual's flexibility and adaptability in coping with his environment (which depend on having the appropriate constructive reactions to external stimuli). The corresponding taste sensation for this circle is salty; the corresponding psychic reaction is fear. Depletion (*inanitas*) of this circle's energy reserves may cause timidity and chronic anxiety and will adversely affect the individual's competence in every sphere of daily life. In the West it has only been since the advent of Sigmund Freud that the close relationship between sexual dysfunction and individual frustration or inadequacy in other areas of life has been studied seriously or scientifically. From a causal-analytic perspective, it may appear (as a rule) that impotence or sexual dysfunction actually *causes* these feelings of anxiety, fearfulness, etc., or, in other words, disappointment in life is the direct result of disappointment in love. From the inductive-synthetic perspective of Chinese medicine, both sexual inadequacy and fear or anxiety may be regarded as manifestations of a single functional disorder. However, since most of us lead relatively uneventful lives and are rarely faced with truly life-threatening situations (or perhaps because sexual inadequacy is modern man's greatest fear), those of us who are suffering from disorders of the function circle of the kidneys might be more aware of (or primarily concerned about) their sexual problems than with fearfulness or anxiety. This is sufficient, in the eyes of Western medicine, to establish a cause-and-effect relationship in which impotence is the primary cause and anxiety the secondary effect.

As far as Chinese medicine is concerned, however, if an individual is

112   suffering from a disorder of the circle of the kidneys, then according to the nature of the situation in which he finds himself (and the nature of the active impulses that make certain demands on his reserves of constructive energy), his "symptoms" may consist of fear or anxiety in one instance and sexual dysfunction in another. Diagnostically the underlying disorder is distinguished by certain quite different characteristics that are independent of the actual situation. Therapeutically it is perhaps worth noting that (in accordance with the axiom that corresponding stimuli will have a beneficial effect on a particular function circle) sexual intercourse might be prescribed (in moderation) as a remedy for fearfulness or anxiety, since it is thought to have a soothing and regulating effect on the circle of the kidneys. And more prosaically, the seasonal and climatic effects associated with winter, the corresponding season, will also have a stimulating effect on this circle. It is also most susceptible to pathological influences (and more responsive to therapeutic intervention) during the hours before midnight. The familiar cyclical litany in the *Suwen* is adjusted accordingly—if a disorder of this circle is not cured during the spring, it will grow worse during the late summer; if the patient can hold out through the fall, "he will arise from his bed in the winter. He should beware of boiling-hot foodstuffs and clothing that has been warmed on the stove." In addition, a disorder of this circle can be expected to go into remission around midnight and then to grow worse again "during the hours of the phase of earth" (i.e., between one and three and again between seven and nine, both A.M. and P.M.). "In the [late] afternoon the patient will find rest."

    Finally, the vocal characteristic that corresponds to this circle (and to the emotion of fear) is groaning or moaning; the *Suwen* also mentions trembling and shivering as being associated with disorders of this circle. The characteristic odor is described as rotten or putrid. The ears are the sensory organs associated with this circle; they are described in the *Suwen* as "the apertures of the circle of the kidneys" (not to be confused with the corresponding bodily orifices, which are the rectum and the urethra).

The Subordinate Official: Function Circle of the Pericardium (Xinbaoluo, Orbis Pericardialis)

Presumably for the sake of symmetry, the pericardial circle was belatedly added as the sixth storage circle, the complementary inner circle to the tricalorium (thus classified as *yin*). It is very sketchily treated in the literature, however, though a number of specific functions are mentioned (which in Western medicine would be variously ascribed to the heart, the lungs, and the circulatory system). It also provides an outlet for the corresponding emotions of joy and pleasure, and, somewhat in the manner of the function circle of the liver, it serves as a kind of self-replenishing reservoir of a form of energy we have denoted *qi genuinum,* a quantity of which we possess at birth and which determines the nature of our "essence" or "inner being."

COMPLEMENTARY FUNCTION CIRCLES

So far we have presented what we hope has been a comprehensive (but certainly far from exhaustive) discussion of the six passage circles, or inner function circles (*intimae*); we have already observed that each of these inner circles has a corresponding outer function circle (*species*), or passage circle, in conjunction with which it is said to form a "functional linkage." This can be regarded as a very close collaboration, and a great many of the orbisiconographic phenomena associated with certain storage circles are also characteristic of the corresponding passage circle. In those cases where it is not even necessary to differentiate between them, they may be treated as a single entity, as we have already done on occasion in the case of the circles of the kidneys and the stomach (*orbes lienalis et stomachi*).

It is also true that a number of diagnostic assertions concerning these passage circles can be indirectly confirmed only by observing the corresponding storage circle. Active *yang* influences are very powerful in themselves, but they become truly definitive only when they can act upon some material object and thus effect certain constructive changes in its makeup. For example, the active component of the *descent* of a falling object from a given height is clearly independent of the nature of the surface on which it is shortly due to land. However, in considering the *effect* of the impact, it matters enormously whether this surface is composed of earth, water, sand, or soil—the nature of the constructive resistance that it offers to the object's descent, or the *yin* component, in other words. (In such a case clearly the term *constructive* should not be taken too literally.) Sometimes the dynamic *yang* component of an event can be determined only if there is a constructive reaction (in which matter is transformed, for example, or the human body undergoes some alteration) involving a complementary functional linkage that shares some of the same characteristics.

Yet there are times when experienced doctors still can distinguish complementary function circles with no difficulty at all because they differ in various important ways, including their associated pulse patterns,

114   impulse points, arterial pathways (by means of the latter two the function circle can be directly influenced with needles or moxa), and certain specific functions. The passage circles also have their own pathology to some extent, since they are subject to disorders that do not affect the complementary storage circles; frequently, however, the disruption of a passage circle will be accompanied by a certain sympathetic delay or retardation in the activities of the corresponding storage circle.

THE PASSAGE CIRCLES (Fu, Orbes Aulici)

In Chapter 11 of the *Suwen* we are informed that the passage circles "transmit and assimilate, store [under pathological conditions], are replenished (*repleti*), but can never be filled up." And, as you may recall, Chapter 47 of the *Lingshu* states that "the six passage circles assimilate liquid and solid nourishment and transmit the active and constructive fluids." Though the meaning of these two passages, wrenched out of context as they are, may still be at least partially obscure, it does seem apparent that, in comparison with the storage circles, the passage circles play a much more active, more markedly *functional* role. The connection between these clearly defined functions and their anatomical namesakes, however, is no more a matter of serious concern than in the case of the storage circles; as we shall see shortly, this appears to be somewhat less true than usual in the case of the two circles of the intestine (*orbes intestinorum*), but in fact the Chinese were not overly interested in what might be called the mechanics of the digestive process until after they had had some exposure to Western notions of anatomy and physiology. There are no *direct* correspondences between these function circles and sensory organs or bodily orifices, psychic reactions, fundamental functions, or storage functions; in general the orbisiconography of the passage circles is less complex and well defined.

Function Circle of the Gall Bladder (Tan, Orbis Felleus)

According to the *Suwen,* "The decisions of all the other eleven circles originate in the circle of gall." The function circle of the gall bladder is accordingly designated as the master-at-arms, "the official in charge of maintaining order" for the total organism, the source of all resolution and determination. In dynamic terms, this function circle regulates the impulses of the other circles themselves (whereas the circulation of the various forms of energy is controlled by the function circles of the heart and the lungs). The circle of the gall bladder is classified as *yang,* of course, and it is the complement of the function circle of the liver. You may have noticed that this circle was also included in the list of supplementary function circles (*paraorbes*) given on page 94; these, again according to the *Suwen,* have their origins in "a constellation of earth," an energy constellation of constructive polarity. The *paraorbes* are thus regarded as function circles that store constructive energy but do not emit or transmit energy of any kind. The circle of the gall bladder is eligible for admission into the ranks of the passage circles only because it is involved in the process of assimilation (but not of the temporary accumulation and transport of liquid and solid nourishment); its ambiguous status is taken into account by means of this twofold classification.

Function Circle of the Small Intestine (Xiaochang, Orbis Intestini Tenuis)

This circle has the task of assimilating and processing the food we eat; more specifically, the finer components are separated from the coarse, the "clear" from the "turbid," and the solid from the liquid, and at this point the process of allocation and distribution begins.

Function Circle of the Stomach (Wei, Orbis Stomachi)

This function circle is pictured by the Chinese as a "city marketplace," or, as we might say, a central reception facility for the nourishment we take in and a kind of transit depot where foodstuffs "of the five taste sensations" (i.e., of every kind) are divided up for distribution. This circle is associated with the transformation phase of earth, and it accordingly plays much the same sort of central intermediary role as does its counterpart, the circle of the spleen, among the storage circles. Primarily, though, it can be regarded as the main reservoir from which the energy derived from the food we eat is conveyed to the other eleven function circles. "Once the energy constellation of the circle of the stomach is allowed to perish, then even the hundred remedies are likely to fail of their effect"—or so we are informed by the *Yizong bidu,* "Compulsory Lectures Drawn from the Medical Tradition." This means, of course, that there is no medicine at all that will be of any use once the harmonious functioning of this circle has been permanently disrupted.

Function Circle of the Large Intestine (Dachang, Orbis Intestini Crassi)

Basically, this circle carries on the task of the circle of the small intestine as described earlier, ensuring the further transformation of nourishment into energy and expediting the transmission of the latter throughout the

116   body. In the concert of the function circles this circle accordingly represents maintenance and continuity.

Function Circle of the Bladder (Pangguang, Orbis Vesicalis)

In Chinese medicine this circle is more picturesquely likened to "the chief city of a district" in which the products of the surrounding countryside—or, in this case, the active and constructive fluids that are the products of the process of assimilation and digestion—are gathered and stored, though they will also undergo further processing, one final transformation, before they are transported elsewhere. Consequently, Chinese medicine attributes a great many more functions to this circle than are customarily ascribed to the urinary bladder in Western medicine (including a number that are associated with the kidneys and the large and small intestines, according to the Western system of correspondences). Functional activity in this region is closely interrelated, however, which means, among other things, that the function circle of the bladder is associated with the circle of the kidneys in a complementary functional linkage.

"The Region of Threefold Warmth" (Sanjiao, Orbis Tricalorii)

The celebrated Chinese doctor Sun Simo (who is said to have died in the year 682 at the age of a hundred) summarized the important attributes of this circle with lapidary succinctness: "The tricalorium has a name but no corporeal form." Other medical texts had at least attempted to specify the location of this anomalous function circle; in the *Lingshu,* for example, the Yellow Prince is made to ask the Count of Qi, "Explain to me now, what is the origin of this threefold warmth." The count replies, "The upper region of warmth begins at the upper aperture of the stomach [called the *cardia* in Western anatomy] and extends upward along with the gullet, through the diaphragm, and then outward into the rib cage. The middle region also begins in the stomach and is located behind the upper region. The lower region extends downward from the ileum [the final section of the small intestine] and pours out its energy into the bladder." Since the time of Sun Simo, however, no subsequent forays into the mysterious realms of anatomy were attempted, and later writers confined themselves to describing the functions associated with this circle.

In the context of the total organism, the tricalorium plays the role of "connective waterway," a kind of thermodynamic Grand Canal that provides the basic medium for the circulation of active and constructive fluids and, in concert with other function circles, is responsible for the regulation of this energy traffic. "It provides the central direction for the energy of all the circles, whether this takes the form of defensive energy (*wei*) or constellational energy (*ying*), whether it acts inside or outside the arterial pathways, on the left or on the right, in the upper or lower regions. If the energy of the threefold region of warmth is uniformly distributed, then the inner [circles] will be in harmony with the outer. Of all the functions that embrace the entire being of the individual and permeate the entire body, of all that bring harmony to the inner and the outer regions, of all that bring to fruition what is on the left-hand side and preserve what is on the right, of all that lead upward and transmit downward, none is more crucial than this one."[4] At any rate, the tricalorium is so described, in highly rhetorical, almost rhapsodic terms, in a treatise titled *Zhongzangjing,* composed sometime during the Sung Dynasty (tenth to thirteenth centuries A.D.). In most of the medical literature, however, this anomalous function circle plays a strictly subordinate role, though it is occasionally invoked in works dealing with sinarteriology (the study of the arterial pathways), where its presence is primarily required for reasons of symmetry.

The tricalorium is also of some interest to the historian of science as an example of the ways in which empirical observation (at various stages of refinement) have been reconciled with the prevailing theoretical paradigm. At first, before the technique of pulse diagnosis had been perfected, Chinese doctors were obliged, for diagnostic purposes, to divide the body into three different "regions of warmth." Each was regarded as the seat or the origin of different vital activities and different forms of individual behavior (the upper region, by the way, extended roughly from the nipples upward, the lower from the navel downward). Then, as the technique of pulse diagnosis became more sophisticated, it became possible to associate a different pulse pattern with each of the function circles, though the concept of the "threefold region of warmth" was never abandoned outright and continued to play a part (sometimes beneficial, sometimes detrimental) in the development of Chinese medical theory. It is perhaps to be regarded as a sign of the maturity of the science of orbisiconography that the tricalorium has been progressively demoted to its current secondary, almost vestigial status (though each of the other function circles is still assigned to a different "region of warmth" in quite straightforward fashion, viz., the circles of the lungs and heart to the upper region, the circles of the spleen, stomach, liver, and gall bladder to the middle region, and the circles of the kidneys, bladder, and large and small intestines to the lower region).

IV

SINARTERIOLOGY

The Doctrine of the Impulse Points and the Arterial Pathways

AS we have seen, Chinese medicine has primarily been identified in the West with acupuncture (and, to a lesser extent, moxibustion) since the European "rediscovery" of China in the seventeenth century. The first published accounts of Chinese medicine, which appeared around the turn of the eighteenth century, were written by Drs. Ten Rhyne and Kaempfer, both of whom had served at the Dutch East India Company's trading station in Japan; these not surprisingly concentrated on the exotic practice of acupuncture. The first Westerner to entertain the possibility that acu-moxa-therapy might be of some benefit was a Frenchman, Félix Vicq-d'Azyr (1748–94), and the Académie des Sciences appointed a commission to investigate this phenomenon for themselves. There is some evidence of sporadic interest in acupuncture in other parts of Europe as well. A professor of medicine at Würzburg, Johann Baptist Friedrich, presented an address describing his own experiments with acupuncture to a convention of German doctors and "natural philosophers" at Frankfurt in 1825; a Swede named Gustav Landgren presented his dissertation on the subject at Uppsala in 1829. Doctors at the Charité Hospital in Berlin undertook a series of experiments with various techniques of acupuncture at about the same time, and the first attempts at electroacupuncture (in which the needles are connected to a "voltaic pile," a primitive form of storage battery) also date from this period.

But serious interest in acupuncture seems to have died down fairly quickly, however, and it is primarily thanks to the individual efforts of a handful of doctors (notably Franz Hübotter and Gerhard Bachmann) that it was not simply allowed to lapse into oblivion during the first half of our own century. Then, as we have already described, the revival of traditional Chinese medicine under the aegis of Mao Zedong was followed in rapid sequence, about twenty years later, by a sudden awakening of Western scientific interest in the newly developed Chinese

122   techniques of acuanalgesia and anesthesia, by the epochal appendectomy of James Reston, and by the worldwide acupuncture boom of the 1970s. It was soon discovered that acupuncture had other applications as well— that it was useful, for example, in treating migraine, neuralgia, toothache, and a great many other bodily ills. Almost without exception, however, Western doctors became accustomed to insert their needles according to a prescribed formula, which was entirely based on the empirical observation that certain disorders appeared to respond favorably when a particular "acupuncture point" (or a combination of points) was stimulated with a needle.

Acu-moxa-therapy, as practiced in the context of systematic Chinese medicine, does not use such empirical formulas; instead the impulse points (*foramina;* singular, *foramen*) to which the needles (or the smoldering moxa leaves) are applied are chosen with the help of diagnostic findings that are entirely determined in accordance with the rational postulates of Chinese medical theory. The theoretical basis for acu-moxa-therapy is furnished by the doctrine of the impulse points and arterial pathways (which we would like to designate, respectively, as foraminology and sinarteriology).

INTRODUCTION TO THE IMPULSE POINTS

Some of the impulse points do have a fixed location, but others manifest themselves only in connection with certain disorders, either in the form of an unusually sensitive, even painful spot accompanied by raised areas, or swellings on the skin. Thus they may be of diagnostic as well as therapeutic significance (since needles may be inserted in these anomalous impulse points in accordance with a diagnosis that has been confirmed by other means). In Chinese the impulse points are called *xue,* which literally means "hole," "aperture," or "cavity"—for which we propose the precise Latin equivalent, *foramen,* which means both a hole or an aperture as well as a recess or cavity. In fact, the impulse points are frequently found in recesses or cavities adjacent to the surface of the body, where they can be palpated (felt) directly by an experienced doctor. There are other impulse points through which the energy that circulates through the body may be released toward the surface, and these may be stimulated with a needle as a means of directly influencing the energy flow. The patient as well as the doctor may be aware of these impulse points, since certain illnesses may cause them to become abnormally sensitive to pain or pressure.

In general the impulse points are divided into three major categories.

1. The *foramina ad hoc*. These are impulse points that the doctor is
   not familiar with and that must, as the name implies, be located
   and treated on a case-by-case basis, either with massage or by the
   insertion of needles.
2. The *foramina extracardinalia*. These are impulse points that the
   doctor is familiar with (since they can be found in everyone in
   the same location) but that are not located on the arterial
   pathways. Several hundred such points have been described in
   the literature so far, and since they have not really been
   incorporated into the rather restricted schematic framework of
   sinarteriology, they are primarily of therapeutic (rather than
   diagnostic) interest.
3. The *foramina cardinalia*. These are impulse points whose locations on the surface of the body have been mapped (over the last
   two millennia) with precise, topographical accuracy and that are
   connected by arterial pathways.

INTRODUCTION TO THE ARTERIAL PATHWAYS

Though the study of the impulse points—foraminology, as we have
termed it—is based purely on clinical experience and is thus an empirical
science, the doctrine of the arterial pathways represents the distillation of
all these empirical data into a rational, theoretical schema. And although
the arterial pathways (most frequently but not very aptly called "meridians" in the Western literature on acupuncture) are conceived of as the
conduits through which the various forms of physiological energy are
transmitted, these pathways in themselves are purely theoretical con-
structs (hypothetical lines, if you will, that connect the empirical "dots"
represented by the impulse points). This is by no means to imply that the
flow of energy along these pathways (i.e., from one point to another)
cannot also be demonstrated empirically. Japanese researcher Yoshio
Manaka has done just that by running a wire between his acupuncture
needles *in situ* (with a semiconductor diode hooked up between them so
that the current could flow in only one direction).[1] This arrangement
permitted Manaka to monitor both the flow of the current and the
therapeutic success of the treatment simultaneously, but such experimental evidence as this serves only to confirm the essential correctness of the
Chinese theoretical model.

The Chinese word we have been translating as "arterial pathway" is
jingmo; mo is equivalent to the Latin *arteria,* which means both "pulse"
and "artery," and *jing* means "course" or "path," among a number of

124   other things (see page 129 for further etymological details). To avoid confusion between *arteria* and *artery,* as that term is used in Western medicine, the standardized nomenclature has added the prefix *sin-* ("Chinese," as in *sinology, sinologue*) to produce *sinarteria* (plural, *sinarteriae*). And since the doctrine of the arterial pathways provides a kind of theoretical superstructure for the empirical study of the impulse points, these two closely related disciplines are generally referred to collectively as *sinarteriology.* Basically each of the twelve function circles is provided with a complementary pair of major arterial pathways (*sinarteriae cardinales*), one for each side of the body. The fact that the entire system is regarded as being symmetrical means that any description of the course or other characteristics of one member of each pair can be assumed to be valid for the other. These "cardinal pathways," as we shall call them, act as extensions of their associated function circles and (in conjunction with a second major class of arterial pathways, the *sinarteriae reticulares,* or "arterial network") help to create the functional linkages by means of which each circle achieves completion and by which the flow of energy and the dynamic harmony between corresponding "inner" (*intima*) and "outer" (*species*) circles are assured. The discussion that follows will concentrate almost exclusively on the classification and the therapeutic and diagnostic significance of this first major class of arterial pathways, the "cardinal pathways," or *sinarteriae cardinales.*[2]

THE CARDINAL PATHWAYS

As we have just seen, each of the *sinarteriae cardinales* is associated with a particular function circle; a cardinal pathway that is associated with a storage circle (*orbis horrealis*) is referred to as a *cardinalis yin,* a cardinal pathway associated with a passage circle (*orbis aulicus*) as a *cardinalis yang.* Each cardinal pathway connects its corresponding passage circle to the storage circle that acts as its complement (in this capacity the pathway may also be designated as a *cardinalis speciei,* since it is associated with an "outer" circle). Each cardinal *yin* pathway helps to connect its associated storage circle to the complementary passage circle (and is thus given the alternative designation *cardinalis intimae,* "inner cardinal"). Note that a function circle is not connected directly to its complement by a single arterial pathway; instead, its corresponding cardinal pathway is connected (indirectly, by means of the network of *sinarteriae reticulares,* "reticular pathways," mentioned earlier) to a complementary pathway of the opposite polarity, which in turn is connected to the complementary circle.

Each of these cardinal pathways begins at one impulse point and ends at another. A more detailed description of the course it takes may refer to any of four different reference points: (1) the trunk, the extremities, or the head; (2) the upper or lower part of the body (with the diaphragm serving more or less as the line of demarcation); (3) the front or the rear of the body; and (4) the actual direction of the energy flow. In general, it may be observed that the cardinal pathways associated with the "upper" storage circles (those of the heart, lungs, and pericardium) run along the *inner* side of the arms—i.e., the upper extremities; those associated with the "lower" storage circles (those of the liver, spleen, and kidneys) run along the *inner* side of the legs. Each of these *cardinales intimae* (i.e., those associated with an "inner," or storage, circle) links up with its complementary *cardinalis speciei* (via the reticular network) at an impulse point either in the fingertips or the tips of the toes. The *cardinales speciei* associated with the circles of the large and small intestines and the tricalorium (complements of the circles of the heart, lungs, and pericardium) run along the *outside* of the arms, and the *cardinales speciei* associated with the circles of the gall bladder, the stomach, and the bladder (complements of the "lower" storage circles) run along the *outside* of the legs. The *cardinales* that run along the arms are designated *cardinales yang* (or *yin*) *manuum,* those that run down through the legs *cardinales yang* (or *yin*) *pedum.* The head, as the uppermost part of the body, is classified as *yang,* and all six of these *cardinales yang* have their "terminus" at an impulse point in the head. The rear of the body is also classified as *yang,* and two of the *cardinales yang pedum* (the exception is the *cardinalis stomachi*) run down the back and sides of the body from head to foot. The *cardinales yin manuum* run from the chest to the hands, and the *cardinales yin pedum* from the chest to the feet. The number of impulse points that lie along the individual pathways may vary a great deal—from a mere nine in the case of the *cardinales cardialis et pericardialis* to as many as sixty-seven in the case of the *cardinalis vesicalis.* These *foramina cardinalia* are numbered consecutively; they also have individual Chinese names (which fortunately need not concern us at the moment). And of much greater concern (therapeutically, at least) than this complex and rather formal business of identifying all the various points and pathways by name is the process of making qualitative distinctions among them; this is done by referring to certain normative conventions, the five transformation phases in particular. As we shall see shortly, such distinctions are extremely useful in providing the doctor with a theoretical framework that enables him to

126   select the appropriate therapy (the point or points at which the needles
or moxa are to be applied) solely on the basis of his initial diagnosis.

THE FIVE INDUCTION POINTS

Strictly speaking, all impulse points are "induction points" by definition—that is, points at which potential changes in the flow of energy may
be induced. However, there are five points that are so called on each of
the twelve cardinal pathways, each one corresponding to one of the five
transformation phases; in this context they may be referred to as the
foramen ligni (transformation phase of wood), *foramen ignis* (fire), *foramen
humi* (earth), *foramen metalli* (metal), and *foramen aquae* (water). These
induction points are all to be found fairly near the endpoints of the
cardinal pathways—in the arms and legs, in other words; they often
represent contiguous impulse points along a particular pathway, though
there may at times be an interval of one or more points between them.
Even so, they are close enough together that the therapist may insert his
needles or apply the moxa in accordance with the classic transformation-
phase sequences described in an earlier section (see pages 68–69).

There is also an extremely well-defined relationship between each of
these five impulse points and a particular pathological state. The
so-called fountain point (*jing, foramen puteale*), which is always to be
found at the tip of a finger or toe, seems to have a special affinity for
congestion of the epigastric region (the upper abdominal region, near the
midline of the body). The second induction point, the "point of effusion"
(*xing, foramen effusorium*), is associated with *calor* and may be stimulated
if fever is present. The third point, the "point of induction" (*shu, foramen
inductorium*), may be stimulated when the body's central equilibrium
(the proper integration of external impulses) has been disturbed, the
symptoms of which include dizziness and pains in the joints. One or
more of the "points of transition" (*jing, foramina transitoria*) may be
stimulated when the normal balance between the inner and outer circles,
intima and *species,* has been disturbed; symptoms include shivering, hot
flashes, shortness of breath, and a number of others. Finally, the "points
of connection" (*he, foramina coiunctoria*), located at the knees or elbows,
are associated with circulatory problems, and problems with retention of
fluids, as well as with diarrhea and incontinence of urine.

Naturally, the doctor's diagnosis in an individual case will determine
which of the twelve points in each group—one for each of the cardinal
pathways—are to be stimulated. And it need hardly be said that the
daunting task of choosing the right impulse points is expedited almost as

much by practical, "hands on" medical experience as by a theoretical 127
mastery of the subject. The foregoing discussion should also make it clear how high a premium is placed on theoretical-model building in Chinese medicine (assuming always that theory is solidly grounded in empirical knowledge).

THE ARTERIAL TERMINALS (FORAMINA NEXORIA)

We have already mentioned that the reticular pathways (*sinarteriae reticulares,* from the Latin *reticulum,* "network") complete the linkage between complementary arterial pathways (and thus between complementary function circles). Thus the complementary *sinarteriae* do not line up directly; as we have seen, each one ends at a terminal impulse point where the flow of energy is transferred or diverted through a reticular pathway to another such point, which serves as the terminus for the complementary arterial pathway. These terminal points are known as *foramina nexoria* (singular, *foramen nexorium;* from the Latin *nexus,* "fastening," "binding"), and they are consequently of great importance in the diagnosis and treatment of any disorder that involves a disruption of this process of energy transfer.

THE GAPS IN THE SYSTEM (FORAMINA RIMICA)

The Latin word *rima* means a "cleft" or "fissure," and these "interstitial points" are located within folds or wrinkles of the skin of the arms and legs, where physiological energy may be allowed to accumulate, resulting in a kind of blockage or congestion. This in turn may result in a particularly stubborn imbalance or disturbance in the flow of energy along that pathway, and these points are often stimulated in cases where the patient's illness proves to be especially stubborn and severe. There is one *foramen rimicum* on each of the cardinal pathways, and an additional four on the *cardinales impares.*

THE DORSAL INDUCTION POINTS (INDUCTORIA DORSALIA)

Altogether there are eighteen impulse points on the back (Latin, *dorsum*), all of which lie along the *cardinalis vesicalis* (the cardinal pathway associated with the function circle of the bladder). These points are of special significance because it is here that the active impulses of all twelve function circles (as well as those of the so-called six bodily regions, which we shall be getting to shortly) can be stimulated most intensively and specifically, and these points are accordingly very useful in treating any

128   disorders that involve the expansive active functions of the various circles.

THE ABDOMINAL "MOBILIZATION POINTS" (CONQUISITORIA ABDOMINALIA)

Essentially these are the *yin* counterparts of the dorsal induction points (hence, they are to be found on the abdomen), which perform a similar office with respect to the constructive aspects of the twelve function circles. The Chinese term for these points is *mu,* which means (like the Latin *conquirire,* from which we have derived our technical term *conquisitorium*) "to assemble (the people) for the purpose of some collective enterprise." The point of this analogy is that all the constructive (i.e., material) resources of a particular function circle are brought to bear on—or, in a word, "mobilized" at—one of these *conquisitoria.* The correlation between the individual points and their respective function circles has been the result of many centuries of clinical investigation— apparently a process in which the requirements of systematic model building have been subordinated to empirical observation, since only three of these points are located on their "own" cardinal pathways (the *conquisitoria pulmonale, hepaticum, et felleum*); six more of these points are located on the *cardinalis renalis,* one on the *cardinalis pulmonalis et stomachi,* and the remaining two are also on the *cardinales hepatica et fellea.*

Here we would like to conclude our discussion of the doctrine of the impulse points, which we embarked on to demonstrate that the practitioner's decision to insert a needle at one or more of these "acupuncture points" is not entirely based on clinical experience but that there is a whole host of theoretical considerations that may also apply. In any truly problematical situation, the doctor can decide only on the basis of his diagnosis in conjunction with his theoretical knowledge whether or not the insertion of a needle at a given point is likely to expedite or to interfere with the healing process. But of course even in China these theoretical and rational considerations are not always given their due, and there, too, the practice of medicine (especially among the "barefoot doctors," paramedics who work primarily in rural areas) frequently relies too heavily on prescribed formulas, a problem that Western medicine (and Western science in general) is equally familiar with. In a case where a particular body of knowledge does rest on a secure theoretical foundation, one sometimes has a tendency to focus one's attention on the practical applications of this knowledge and to forget

about theory altogether. This does not mean, of course, that the
theoretical foundations of this knowledge have ceased to exist or that
they are no longer of any particular importance.

DIAGNOSTIC PROFILE OF THE CARDINAL PATHWAYS

After the courses of the cardinal pathways have been mapped and the
impulse points charted and classified (an exercise we will be attempting
shortly), the next step is to provide a description of the characteristic
symptoms that manifest themselves when the normal functions of the
cardinal pathways are disrupted. (This is the primary way in which these
functions can be rectified therapeutically—when the circulation of
energy along the pathways is suspended or disturbed.) This will also
complete our discussion of the orbisiconography of the individual
function circles (the orbisiconography customarily make some mention
of the corresponding cardinal pathways for each circle). It should also be
borne in mind, as in the immediately preceding sections, that since the
cardinal pathways are arrayed symmetrically in pairs (with respect to the
midline of the body), the following descriptions of the individual
cardinales hold true for both the right- and left-hand members of a pair.

As mentioned earlier, the Chinese word we have been translating as
"pathway" is *jing,* which originally referred to the warp (the lengthwise
threads) that gives shape and solidity (*definition,* in other words) to a
piece of woven fabric. By extension, *jing* also came to denote anything
definitive or authoritative, a "classic" (e.g., the celebrated *Yijing*); in the
medical literature, however, *jing* was primarily used as a verb that meant
"to lead along certain lines" or "to set a particular course for something"
and thus was admirably suited to describing the functions of the arterial
pathways that transmit the body's physiological energy along a predetermined course. The *sinarteriae reticulares* (the "reticular pathways" that
connect complementary cardinal pathways to one another) are called *luo*
in Chinese, which literally means "to tie up" or "fasten," "to make into
a net," "to catch in a net." (The Latin word *reticulum,* originally "a string
bag" or the like, is frequently used as a scientific term to refer to a
"network" of any kind.)

The Cardinalis Hepatica

This cardinal pathway, associated with the function circle of the liver,
has its origin directly below the nail of the big toe, runs up the inside of
the leg, detours around the genitals, then heads up the lower central

130   section of the abdomen (the hypogastrium) and veers off to the left (or right) near the stomach to a terminal impulse point on either side of the body, just below the diaphragm. Altogether there are fourteen impulse points along the *cardinalis hepatica.*

The symptoms associated with disruptions of the normal circulation of energy along this pathway include: pains that restrict one's ability to bend at the waist; abdominal swellings (in women); dry throat and mouth; pale or muddy complexion; a feeling of fullness in the chest and upper abdominal region (epigastrium); belching or vomiting; abdominal pains (perhaps including colic); dyspepsia (interruption of the normal process of digestion); diarrhea (or constipation); and incontinence (or retention) of urine. (The widely divergent nature of these last two groups of symptoms may be explained by the fact that a disruption in the normal function of a cardinal pathway may produce either a local surplus or a deficiency of energy.)

The Cardinalis Fellea

This is the cardinal pathway associated with the circle of the gall bladder, the complement of the circle of the liver. It begins its journey near the outer corner of the eye, follows a complicated course around the outside of the head (which includes some twenty impulse points along the way), then down the nape of the neck, over the shoulders, past the arms, and then describes a zigzag pattern down the side of the trunk and the outside of the leg, finally reaching its terminus in the fourth toe. Altogether there are forty-four impulse points along this cardinal pathway.

The relevant symptoms include: a bitter taste in the mouth, sighing and pausing frequently to catch one's breath, muscular pains around the rib cage, and difficulty in bending at the waist or rotating the upper body. Symptoms of more serious disorders may include a pallid, muddy, or dull complexion, emaciation, a burning sensation along the outside of the legs, pains in the legs and joints, swelling of the lymph nodes, spontaneous outbreaks of sweating, shivering, and finally, malaria. It should not be too surprising that these first two lists contain two of the same symptoms (pallor or a muddy complexion), since these two *cardinales* are associated with complementary circles whose functions (and dysfunctions) are closely related.

However, there are also cases in which comparable symptoms might seem to imply a functional connection that does not exist. Individual symptoms considered in isolation are of no great significance in themselves; they must always be interpreted in conjunction with all other available diagnostic signals. A pale face, for example, may just be a transitory reaction (a sign of a sleepless night, perhaps, or an emotional shock) and not really a symptom of an illness at all. The accurate observation and collective interpretation of these diagnostic signs is the *sine qua non* of the Chinese doctor's art and a process we shall frequently be referring to in our discussion of Chinese diagnosis.

The Cardinalis Cardialis

The pathway associated with the function circle of the heart has only nine impulse points along its entire length, fewer than any other. The first of these is located a little in front of the armpit, and from there the *cardinalis cardialis* continues along the inside of the arm and across the palm of the hand, terminating in the tip of the little finger.

Disturbances in the energy flow along this pathway may produce a variety of symptoms, including a dry throat and an intense thirst (not necessarily symptomatic in themselves, of course, unless accompanied by the following), cardiac pains, bruising or discoloration of the skin accompanied by numbness in the underarm region, blurred vision, pains in the area of the rib cage and in the ribs themselves, and pains in or sensitive patches on the palms of the hands.

The Cardinalis Intestini Tenuis

This pathway, associated with the small intestines, begins directly below the nail of the little finger and runs over the ball of the hand and the outside of the arm to the elbow and the shoulder. From there it follows a jagged course over to the collarbone, then upward to an impulse point just below the hinge of the jawbone. Here it splits into two branches, one of which terminates in the cheek, the other of which continues upward to the corner of the eye and thence finally to the ear. Altogether there are nineteen impulse points along this pathway.

Symptoms of related functional disorders include neck pains as well as pain accompanied by swelling of the muscles of the neck, difficulty in turning one's head from side to side, pain and stiffness in the shoulders, and a feeling of extreme weakness in the upper arm. Finally, there may also be a number of additional symptoms that are associated with a *dyscrasia*—in other words, an abnormal imbalance of some physiological element (in this case, of constructive fluids); these include impaired vision and hearing, swellings and pains in the area in and around the

132   lower jaw (pains may also radiate downward through the neck and shoulder blades toward the armpit).

The Cardinalis Lienalis

The cardinal pathway associated with the function circle of the spleen has its origin directly beneath the nail of the big toe and runs up the inside of the leg and past the groin into the abdominal cavity, where it is connected directly with the circle of the spleen as well as indirectly with the function circle of the stomach. The *cardinalis lienalis* splits into two branches, one of which continues upward from the stomach and through the diaphragm to the heart; the other also passes through the diaphragm and the outside (i.e., the right or left side) of the chest to a point below the collarbone, where it veers inward and runs up inside the neck to the root of the tongue. Altogether there are twenty-one impulse points along this pathway.

Symptoms of the related functional disorders may include swelling and sensitivity of the root of the tongue, nausea after meals, stomach pains, swelling of the lower abdominal region (hypogastrium), belching (particularly if there is some alleviation of these latter symptoms after the passing of stool or flatus); generalized physical exhaustion, and a feeling of lassitude. Additional symptoms may include motor problems, circulatory problems (including abnormal coldness of the hands and feet) and cardiac pains, diarrhea or constipation (or other intestinal disorders), retention of urine, jaundice, sleeplessness, swellings along the path of the *cardinalis lienalis* on the inside of the legs (particularly around the thigh or the knee), and paralysis of the big toe.

The Cardinalis Stomachi

This is the only *cardinalis yang* pathway whose course takes it down over the chest and belly rather than down the back. It begins by the nostrils, curves upward to a point below the eyes, then turns downward, toward the corner of the mouth and the chin, where it splits into two branches, one of which doubles back along the lower jaw, past the ear, and up to the hairline at the temple. The other branch runs down the neck to the collarbone, where it turns outward (to the left or right) and runs down along the chest, through the nipple, and down the belly to the edge of the pubic hair. There it turns outward once more in the groin region, runs down the front of the thigh, the knee, and the shin, and terminates in the second toe. The *cardinalis stomachi* has forty-five impulse points in all, more than most of the other cardinal pathways.

Pathological symptoms that are associated with disruption of the flow of energy along this pathway include shivering and groaning in particular, along with frequent sneezing. The patient's complexion is described as dark or swarthy. In the early stages of this illness the patient may feel an aversion to other human beings as well as to fire and warmth. In its more critical stages, the patient's entire body may swell up, accompanied by rumblings in the stomach and sometimes by an outbreak of boils and twisted or contorted limbs as well. The *cardinalis stomachi* is also subject to all the various disorders that may result from a deficiency in the circulation of *xue,* which, as you may recall, is defined as "individual-specific constructive energy." These may include malaria; high fever; violent rages; abnormal outbreaks of sweating; a cold with a stopped-up nose; nosebleeds; chapped or split lips; hoarseness accompanied by a swelling of the neck; dropsy; pains in and swellings of the knee joint, in the chest, and around the breastbone as well as in certain parts of the legs; and paralysis of (or at least inability to use) the middle finger. An abundant supply of *xue,* on the other hand, may produce a burning sensation in the abdominal region, and a surplus will result in an overly efficient digestion accompanied by frequent and abnormal hunger pangs. The urine turns bright yellow. A mild energy deficiency may produce a cold sensation in the abdominal region accompanied by shivering and in more serious cases by gastroenteritis as well.

The Cardinalis Pulmonalis

This is one of the shorter cardinal pathways, with only eleven impulse points along its entire length. The pathway associated with the function circle of the lungs begins its course in the middle of the stomach region and turns inward, toward the interior of the body and its indirect functional linkup with the circle of the large intestine. Then it executes an abrupt U-turn slightly below the navel and heads upward as far as the neck, then turns outward toward the shoulder (where its first impulse point is located) and finally runs down along the inside of the arm to the tip of the thumb.

Symptoms associated with dysfunctions of this cardinal pathway include congestion (*repletio*) of the function circle of the lungs—in diagnostic terms, this refers to bronchitis or chronic or acute inflammation of the bronchioles (the tubes that connect the bronchi with the alveoli) as well as coughing, shortness of breath, and asthmatic attacks. The patient may also experience pains in the forearm. A surplus of energy in the function circle of the lungs may cause pains in the

134   shoulders or the shoulder blades, as well as the standard cold symptoms accompanied by spontaneous outbreaks of sweating and urinary incontinence. Other symptoms of energy surplus in this function circle resemble those of the flu—hoarseness, stopped-up nose, and rough or stertorous breathing through the mouth and nose. A deficiency of energy in the circle of the lungs may cause pains in the shoulders and back, shivering, shortness of breath, and discoloration of the urine.

The Cardinalis Intestini Crassi

The cardinal pathway associated with the function circle of the large intestine is a *cardinalis yang,* and as such it begins its course beneath the nail of the index finger and travels up the outside of the arm and the shoulder to the upper back directly below the nape. It divides into two branches at the shoulder blade; the upper branch runs along the side of the neck and ends at an impulse point on the cheek, near the nostril. The lower branch heads downward and into the interior of the body, where it joins the *orbis intestini crassi* in the vicinity of the large intestine. There are twenty impulse points altogether on this pathway.

Associated symptoms include toothache and swelling of the neck. This pathway is also susceptible to dyscratic disorders (in this case brought about by an imbalance in the composition of the blood), the symptoms of which may include yellowing of the whites of the eyes, dry mouth, stopped-up nose, nosebleeds, and hoarseness. The patient may experience pains in the shoulders (as well as in the thumbs or index fingers). An excess of energy in the circle of the large intestine may result in localized swellings along the path of the *cardinalis intestini crassi.* Shivering and a persistent chill (the inability to warm up properly) are taken as signs that the energy reserves of this circle have been depleted.

The Cardinalis Renalis

The cardinal pathway that is associated with the function circle of the kidneys has its origin on the outer edge of the little toe; from there it runs through an impulse point on the sole of the foot, around the ankle, and then—as a *cardinalis yin* pathway—up along the inside of the leg, up the belly (passing directly by the navel) and the chest, terminating at the collarbone. The *cardinalis renalis* joins the function circle of the kidneys in the interior of the body and links up indirectly with the function circle of the bladder. Altogether it has twenty-seven impulse points.

Dysfunctions or disruption of the energy flow in this pathway are characterized by the following symptoms: loss of appetite (accompanied by a hungry or empty feeling), harsh breathing, and coughing (sometimes the sputum may be flecked with blood). The patient's complexion is described as dark and glistening. He may see black spots or bright flashes before his eyes when he stands up; this may be accompanied by a fluttering heartbeat, or an arrhythmia. The symptoms of energy exhaustion (*inanitas*) of this function circle include fearfulness and anxiety; the patient may suffer from chills and have a very rapid pulse rate. He may feel pains in his arms and legs; there may even be restricted mobility. The tongue will feel hot and dry; the throat will be sore and inflamed. Eventually the patient may suffer from cardiac pains and depression. Additional symptoms include jaundice, diarrhea, and back pain. The patient will also feel an urgent need for rest and peace and quiet.

The Cardinalis Vesicalis

As we have seen, the cardinal pathway associated with the function circle of the bladder has more impulse points than any other—sixty-seven in all, which includes the eighteen *inductoria dorsalia*. The *cardinalis vesicalis* begins its course near the inside corner of the eye and travels upward, over the forehead, the dome of the skull, and down to the nape of the neck, where it splits into two branches that run parallel to the backbone, then down over the buttocks and the back of the thigh and that are finally reunited at the knee joint. From here the *cardinalis vesicalis* runs down the fleshy part of the calf, around the outside of the ankle, over the instep, and terminates in the little toe.

The corresponding symptoms include severe and persistent headaches (particularly if the pain is concentrated at the back of the head) and a peculiar feeling of pressure in the eyes, as if they were being pushed out of their sockets, and back pain centering in the backbone itself. The patient will also have a localized sense of muscular fatigue or weakness in the lumbar region and stiffness in the hip and knee joints. In general, any sort of disorder that affects the muscles involved in locomotion may be considered a symptom of a dysfunction in this cardinal pathway.

The Cardinalis Pericardialis

The cardinal pathway associated with the pericardium, the sac that surrounds the heart, begins its course in the chest, slightly to the right (or left) of the nipple, and loops upward toward the chin. As a *yin* pathway it runs down over the biceps, the inside of the forearm, and the palm of the hand to the tip of the middle finger. It links up with the *cardinalis*

136   *tricalorii* in the interior of the body and has only nine impulse points along its entire length.

Symptoms associated with dysfunctions of the *cardinalis pericardialis* include hot flashes or sharp, burning pains in the area of the heart, muscular spasms and cramps around the elbow and in the forearm, and swellings in the shoulders. The patient may experience a feeling of tension or compression in the rib cage, accompanied by heart palpitations. The patient's complexion is described as ruddy or bright red, and he may occasionally suffer from momentary blackouts or paroxysms of wild, inappropriate laughter. Additional symptoms include depression, cardiac pains, and a burning sensation in the palms of the hands.

The Cardinalis Tricalorii

The cardinal pathway associated with the "threefold region of warmth" begins its course at a point directly below the nail of the ring finger and, as a *yang* pathway, continues over the back of the hand and the outside of the arm to the shoulder. Then it proceeds up the neck to a point just below the earlobe, where it splits into two branches. One of these runs across the temple to the outside corner of the eyelid; the other continues in the opposite direction to pick up three more impulse points behind the ear. Altogether there are twenty-three impulse points along this pathway; it joins the threefold region of warmth and links up with the *cardinalis pericardialis* in the interior of the body.

Dysfunctions of the *cardinalis tricalorii* are characterized by deafness, absentmindedness, disorientation, and painful constriction of the throat; many disorders that are associated with an excess or a deficiency of *qi* (active energy) may also affect this pathway, and their symptoms include spontaneous outbreaks of sweating, swollen calves, and pain in the eyelids and the other regions of the body that are traversed by the *cardinalis tricalorii,* especially the ears.

SUMMING IT ALL UP: THE DIAGNOSIS

As we have seen, it is characteristic of Chinese medicine that a single symptom may be associated with a number of different disorders. Part of the reason for this is the constitutional vagueness of language; e.g., all sorts of different pains are referred to as "headache." There are also a great many different disorders whose presence may be evinced by these various "headaches." It is the task of the diagnostician to evaluate the competing claims, so to speak, of all these different disorders by means of a comprehensive review of all the symptoms that had presented themselves at the time of the diagnosis. Only this will enable him to decide which of these disorders—hence, which of these various types of "headache"—the patient is suffering from. Consequently there cannot be said to be a single impulse point, or even a combination of points, that must be stimulated to cure a headache. Instead, the doctor must make this decision purely on the basis of his Chinese diagnosis; it may be, for example, that needles or moxa would not be recommended, and some other approach—a herbal remedy, perhaps—must be attempted instead.

Sinarteriology and the systematic description of the arterial pathways ("meridians") is the one aspect of Chinese medicine that is most accurately presented in the existing literature on the subject. However, we are not concerned with providing the reader with a practical "acupuncture map" but rather with a basic presentation of the theoretical principles and the sort of diagnostic (empirical) observations by which a Chinese doctor is guided in formulating his own diagnosis and in selecting the particular impulse points that are to be stimulated with acu-moxa-therapy. Accordingly we shall make no attempt to describe or chart the courses of the remaining arterial pathways; the interested reader is referred to the Notes for this chapter at the end of the book.[3]

V

DIAGNOSIS

The Chinese Concept of Illness

THE simplest and most accurate definition of this concept might be "a departure from or disturbance in orthopathy (*zheng*)," and, as we have seen, orthopathy is a concept that can be just as accurately if less elegantly defined as "proceeding along a straight path." Orthopathy does not just mean "the state of having nothing wrong with you"; rather it refers specifically to a function that is operating at an optimal level. Suppose, for example, that a greenhouse full of tropical plants is intended to be kept at a constant temperature of 75°F; either a higher or a lower temperature would be detrimental to the welfare of the plants, and the greenhouse has accordingly been equipped with a small heating system that enables the temperature to be regulated very precisely. In such a case, the gardener who looks after such a system would not really need to consult a thermometer that was marked off in degrees but could make do with an indicator with a single red line representing 75°F and a pointer. Any other position of the pointer, above or below the red line, would indicate a departure from optimal functional effectiveness—from orthopathy, in a word—and the system would have to be adjusted accordingly. However, it is important to recall that the position of the pointer, of course, tells us nothing about the *cause* of any particular deviation from the optimum, and we can readily imagine that almost any number of physical, mechanical, and climatic factors might be capable of inducing a temporary state of "heteropathy" in the greenhouse, including anything from a clogged fuel line to a broken pane of glass to an abrupt change in temperature of a degree or two—even perhaps to the sun suddenly coming out from behind a cloud.

An individual human being—and in accordance with the Chinese view of things, we would prefer not to use expressions like "the human body" or "the human organism"—is an incredibly sensitive and complicated system (infinitely more so than a greenhouse or even a delicate

142   tropical plant), which means that the number of factors that can cause functional deviations from a state of orthopathy is incalculably large. We are not just speaking of every sound, every beam of light, every cosmic ray, every fluctuation in temperature or humidity—of every external impulse, in short—but also of intrinsic, "free-floating," and unpredictable mental and emotional impulses, thoughts, and memories. (Consider for a moment the sort of startling physiological effects—including cardiac arrest—that may be brought about by the spontaneous recollection of an emotionally charged experience, no matter whether it was a moment of ecstasy, of outrage, or a humiliation, and no matter that the man or woman within whom this emotional tempest is unleashed has not been exposed to any other pathological influence.) And finally there are also social factors—the mood and the conditions that prevail in a particular human environment, not to mention the often very profound and pernicious influences of certain "environmental" stimuli in the form of manmade radiation and chemical contaminants.

In the case of a relatively crude mechanical system like a heating system, it is generally enough just to keep it running right—functioning at its optimal efficiency—and if there is a breakdown or a disturbance of some kind, it would be sensible to locate the cause of this breakdown and try to set it right, since not all that many things can go wrong with such a system. And when we are confronted instead with the literally countless number of factors that may affect the optimal functioning of an enormously complex system like an individual human being, it may still be advisable to investigate the *known* causes of such dysfunctions (particularly if these have been established on the basis of two thousand years of clinical experience) and try, as before, to put them right. This is especially true if this disruption of orthopathy has persisted long enough to have left unmistakable physical traces on the bodily substrate— engrams, as they are sometimes called—and in fact it is illusory and entirely futile to proceed in such a fashion if either the empirical knowledge or such physical evidence is lacking. Yet in just such a case as this, it is not only advisable but actually necessary, from a medical standpoint, to try to identify the nature of the dysfunction with the greatest possible accuracy (to pinpoint the extent as well as the direction of the indicator's deviation from its optimal reading, in other words). *This and nothing else is the real task of Chinese diagnostic medicine.*

The purpose and intent of this diagnostic method can be further resolved into these separate components: (1) It identifies a disruption of or a departure from orthopathy in an unambiguous, rational, rigorous, as well as reproducible and verifiable manner. This always involves (2) a precise determination of the *direction* of this deviation from a functional optimum (an unambiguous qualitative assertion, in other words, that invokes certain normative conventions). Finally, this diagnostic process also involves (3) making certain decisions about the nature and identity of the pathological agent that has brought about this deviation *in the case of the individual who is the subject of this diagnosis*. The identification of these agents of disruption or dysfunction is largely the concern of the *individual* diagnosis, in other words. Let us choose for our hypothetical agent a common substance like vinegar, for example, to see how this might be the case. If we could persuade a group of test subjects to ingest a quantity of vinegar that was ten times greater than they were accustomed to, every day, then it would not be too much longer before most of them would start to experience subjective and then objective distress and dysfunction. There would be a small group of subjects, however, who could tolerate this massive intake of vinegar without showing any signs of distress; under certain circumstances they might even call out for more. And, by the same token, there would be a third group of subjects who could not even tolerate a "normal" quantity of vinegar in their food; even a drop or two applied to the skin could produce a distinct, or even a violent, abreaction.

Clearly there is something going on in each of these latter two cases that might reasonably be regarded as a proper subject for diagnostic investigation, even in a case where the suspected "pathological agent" is a generally unremarked and unremarkable substance like vinegar. The methods that would be employed in a Chinese diagnosis differ primarily from the causal-analytic procedures of Western medicine in this respect—they would not involve any chemical or material investigation into the composition of the suspected agent itself, nor of the various bodily secretions of the subject, beginning with the products of the urinary and digestive tracts. However, an attempt would be made to provide an exact and *unambiguous* description of the degree to which (and the direction in which) the consumption of or physical contact with this substance has brought about a deviation from orthopathy in this individual case; this description would make use of certain normative conventions, beginning with the so-called eight leading criteria (which we will be discussing shortly) as applied to the disciplines of orbisiconography and sinarteriology, as well as the pulse diagnostic. And, as we have seen in our earlier discussions of these two disciplines, this involves the collection of all the data relevant to the individual patient, including

144   physical observations such as the condition of the tongue or the skin, with due considerations for other symptoms that are purely functional, such as sleeplessness, sensory impairment or disorientation, digestive disorders, abnormal secretions of sweat, and a great deal else besides. In the process of differential diagnosis (which simply means of distinguishing between different disorders that may present a number of similar symptoms), the experienced diagnostician may also evaluate the significance of a great many phenomena that the patient (or any uninstructed layperson) would be unaware of or would be unable to draw any useful conclusions from; this would include certain deductions about the state of individual function circles and impulse points, the iconography of certain pulse points, the relative states of the surface coating and the muscular blade of the tongue, etc.

DESCRIPTIVE CONSIDERATIONS

The diagnostic process is based on four main procedures: visual inspection of the patient, which would include the "tongue diagnostic" just mentioned; questioning the patient directly; evaluating the quality of the patient's voice and the patient's characteristic odor (regarded as a single procedure for purposes of classification); and finally touching, or "palpating," the patient's body (which primarily involves feeling the various pulse points). Superficially the four procedures practiced by Chinese doctors seem largely identical to the initial stages of a consultation with an old-fashioned family doctor in the West, who would invariably look at the patient's tongue, ask a few questions, take his pulse, and poke and prod him in various places. The objects of their investigations, however, are entirely different. A Western doctor might palpate his patient to detect an enlargement of the liver or a localized sensitivity to pressure that may result from some drastic somatic alteration (notoriously, of course, an inflamed appendix). The Chinese doctor is more directly concerned with his patient's reaction to the pressure of his hand, and the decisive question here is whether the pain is increased (a *yang* symptom) or alleviated (a *yin* symptom) by the application of pressure.

Apart from these basic differences of outlook and approach (essentially, the difference between causal-analytic and inductive-synthetic), there is one other important difference between these two diagnostic systems. A Western doctor who observes his patient's pale face, heavily coated tongue, swollen eyes, and thin, scratchy voice will obviously conclude that his patient is sick (and may even recognize what is wrong with him as well). However, if he should base his diagnosis on these observations, he would do so purely in an empirical way—without attempting to elaborate this experientially acquired knowledge into a scientific system and to evaluate all future such diagnoses accordingly. He may frequently be able to explain why his patient's complexion is greenish-gray or why the patient feels generally run down and debilitated, but these explanations are so generalized (i.e., they apply to so many different disorders) that they are relatively meaningless in terms of scientific Western medicine. To present his case scientifically, a Western doctor's diagnosis must involve the search for "pathogens" and reduced blood-sugar levels, the interpretations of X rays, and blood-sedimentation rates.

With a Chinese doctor the situation is quite different. In the first place, the relevant empirical data are gathered in accordance with a scientific system. (This does not mean that every case presents him with a fresh scientific puzzle to unravel, since he can diagnose most routine or trivial illnesses entirely on the basis of experience, just as his Western colleague would.) What it does mean is that all the experientially acquired data about his patient that is accessible to him (i.e., that can be observed externally) are continually integrated into the theoretical system of Chinese medical science and are evaluated accordingly. Many Western doctors, who naturally lack the requisite experience with this sort of medicine as well as the necessary cultural and linguistic background, can come to appreciate Chinese medicine only by means of a rational initiation into this new scientific system. And the correlation of certain empirical characteristics of a patient's appearance or behavior by normative conventions (e.g., the correlation of shallow breathing with taciturnity, or the designation of a pale face or a particular pulse pattern as *"yin* symptoms") is indeed a rational means of organizing a merely empirical body of knowledge (and is therefore not a skill that is immediately available to everyone but depends instead on the specialized knowledge of a doctor who has been educated for the particular purpose of performing this task).

PARALLELS WITH WESTERN BIOLOGICAL SCIENCES

At this stage in his initiation, though, a Western observer might well be tempted to wonder if by proceeding in this direction Chinese medicine could ever arrive at a comprehensive pathology (that is to say, a systematic *taxonomy,* or classification system) of human functional disorders. Skeptics would do well to remember that Western biology was once faced with similar obstacles in its early attempts to provide a

146   descriptive classification system that embraced all living creatures. Harvard zoologist Ernst Mayr has described the original dimensions of the problem in these terms:

> The multiplicity of forms in living nature is overwhelming. More than a million animal species and half a million plant species have already been described; estimates of the number of living creatures that have been systematically described vary between two and three million. If a total of half a billion is suggested for the extinct species, this would be in accordance with the available facts. Each of these species may assume different forms, depending on age, sex, the season, morphological or other variants. This formidable diversity could never be dealt with if it could not be ordered and classified.[1]

But thanks to the binomial classification system that was eventually adopted by Western botanists and zoologists, one need not be a highly trained naturalist to discern an underlying pattern in the extraordinary diversity of life on earth, and with the help of a field guide or two, the interested layman can readily identify most of the plant and animal species he is likely to encounter along a woodland trail or in an Alpine meadow.

It is easy enough to see how a system of this kind might succeed in imposing order on the vast diversity of human diseases, and that this might be done in any number of ways (including the Chinese way). In fact, there are a number of parallels between Chinese medicine and Western taxonomy. Taxonomy, as such, is not concerned with *causes;* it is not concerned with finding out why swans are white but rather with deciding that a certain kind of big white bird is called a swan (or, rather, *Cygnus olor*). Chinese medicine also distinguishes seasonal varieties of certain illnesses, and in general, Chinese doctors classify (that is, diagnose) their patients in much the same way that Western biologists might classify birds or plants. A Chinese doctor who observes a patient's dirty-white complexion (a *yin* symptom) is in much the same position as a biologist who has heard someone talking about a "big white bird." But in either case the process of classification can proceed very rapidly on the basis of a handful of observed characteristics (as the vast, almost infinite multitude of *observable* characteristics just as rapidly become irrelevant or dwindle into insignificance). It is interesting to note that (for the most part) the taxonomist is not guided by complex anatomical or physiological considerations but by an orderly, diminishing series of relatively straightforward external characteristics of appearance and behavior. His special-ized knowledge enables him to decide which of these characteristics are important and which are irrelevant, until finally he is able to decide quite confidently that he is face to face with the mute swan (*Cygnus olor*)—in much the same way that the Chinese doctor comes to decide that his patient is suffering from a disorder called *"ventus* heteropathy" (for the moment we need not concern ourselves too much with what this means).

It is perhaps also worth noting (though this is not directly relevant to this process of classification) that scientists who study animal behavior (ethologists) are in the habit of collecting data on "macrocosmic" phenomena that can be correlated very closely with certain patterns of behavior. This is most apparent, of course, in the seasonal mating, nesting, and migratory habits of a great many species of birds, but it has also been observed that the "circadian rhythms" or "internal clocks" of a wide variety of birds, animals, even insects and invertebrates, as well as human beings, appear to be set in accordance with the cycle of the seasons, the relative lengths of day and night, the rhythm of the tides, or the phases of the moon. This would come as no great surprise to the authors of the *Suwen,* who, as we saw earlier in our discussion of orbisiconography, devoted a great deal of attention to the diurnal and seasonal variations in the normal course of an illness.

We have also seen that observation of human behavior plays an important role in Chinese medicine as well. However, the behavior patterns that are associated with certain disorders are not characterized, as they tend to be in the West, as "abnormal" or as outright "behavioral disorders," and thus as *secondary illnesses* in their own right whose causes have to be investigated. (This point is worth stressing, among other reasons, because this is only a step away from labeling the patient himself as "deviant" or "abnormal.") In Chinese medicine, on the other hand, such behavior is simply regarded as *normal behavior for sick people* and thus as merely an additional symptom of the primary disorder. Of these two approaches certainly the second is much more in accordance with recent (though admittedly provisional) findings in the realm of social psychology and human ethology.

The fact that there is no sharp philological distinction between the ordinary Chinese language and "the language of science" should not mislead us into thinking that Chinese medicine has not evolved a comprehensive scientific vocabulary that is intelligible only to a specially trained practitioner. Medical terms like *dongmo* ("moving pulse," *pulsus mobilis*) or *huamo* ("slippery pulse," *pulsus lubricius*) are scarcely more

148   meaningful to the Chinese layman than a technical term from the International Scientific Vocabulary like *Müllerian mimicry* would be to the uninstructed Westerner. (This refers, by the way, to the fact that certain edible species of butterflies [e.g.] tend to mimic the bright colors of inedible or even venomous species to ward off potential predators.)

We should like to point out one final parallel between Chinese medicine and Western behavioral science (though here *behavior* is used in a slightly different sense, to mean the object of experiment—or therapy—rather than simple observation). We all know that animals' primarily instinctive responses to certain stimuli enable scientists not only to predict but also to elicit certain kinds of behavior at will. In much the same way, a Chinese doctor can predict on the basis of his diagnosis which therapeutic stimuli will cause the system of the function circles to give the desired response—namely, systemic motion in the direction of orthopathy, of good health. Thus (with the full knowledge and cooperation of the patient, of course) he applies needles or moxa to particular impulse points, prescribes certain breathing exercises or medications or a particular dietary regime, and so forth. Chinese medicine regards the process of healing from a uniquely humanistic perspective; thus it is not conceived of as a sequence of biochemical events but rather as a pattern of human behavior that is fully in accord with prevailing external and environmental conditions.

The Differences Between Western and Chinese Diagnostic Medicine

BEFORE we proceed any farther with the subject of Chinese diagnosis, we would like to say a word or two about the various hybrid forms of Chinese and Western medicine—most of which have passed unchallenged under the name "Chinese medicine" in the West, particularly if their practitioners have acquired their skills in Hong Kong, Taiwan, or the People's Republic itself. All of these medical hybrids are distinguished by the fact that they employ the techniques of acu-moxa-therapy, but only in accordance with a Western-style diagnosis or (failing a positive diagnostic finding) as part of a strictly empirical attempt to correlate the disappearance of certain symptoms with the stimulation of a particular group of impulse points with needles or moxa.

The results of these experiments are often (though not invariably) successful but not scientifically verifiable—in much the same way that certain disorders seem to respond favorably to treatment at spas and mineral springs even though no scientific explanation for this is forthcoming. As far as the patient is concerned, of course, the success of the cure is far more important than scientific rigor or the soundness of its theoretical underpinnings, but the doctor should presumably have some interest in discovering where his findings can be confirmed scientifically (i.e., whether they are reproducible) and where they cannot. The scope of medical practice in China has been increased enormously over the past century or so by means of practical and theoretical contributions from the West; here at last Chinese medicine (which includes diagnostic medicine and medical theory as well as therapeutic technique) is finally in a position to return the favor.

THE ROLE OF QUANTITATIVE DATA

A Western doctor arrives at a diagnosis essentially by comparing the quantitative data he has collected about his patient with a corresponding

150   set of normal values. He takes his patient's pulse and temperature, measures his blood pressure, and counts his red and white corpuscles. He may subject the patient's body to stress in certain precisely predetermined ways to measure its reaction (tests for diabetes, for example, or circulatory "stress tests"). At first glance there may seem to be little difference between this aggregation of normal values—the Western standard of good health—and the Chinese concept of orthopathy. In fact, the difference is considerable. All of this quantitative information (including the normal values) is just a series of analytical assertions—isolated statements of fact, in other words, that are not correlated with other data and thus are general rather than specific in character. "Isolated" means in this case that these values were obtained independently of one another (thus without consideration for—or in other words, excluding—all other available information) and that for the most part they are only correlated with other measurable data about an individual patient (i.e., statements for which a causal explanation might be sought) in a way that is imprecise, superficial, and even seemingly quite illogical. A pulse rate of 120 may be cause for alarm—unless the "patient" has just finished a ten-mile run, in which case it is perfectly normal. A doctor can decide whether a given diagnostic finding is "normal" or "pathological" only by taking all other relevant factors into account, and these normal quantitative values are not necessarily relevant to a given individual case (since they are based on a statistical cross section of a very large group of similar or comparable cases). In this sense, at least, orthopathy is the precise opposite of quantitative "normality."

We have already seen that orthopathy is maintained—and thus can be disrupted—by an almost infinite variety of dynamic factors, many of which are extremely volatile, and that this constantly shifting dynamic equilibrium determines whether or not an individual feels well and is capable of leading a normal, active life. This implies, given the complexity and instability of the situation, that the individual himself should ultimately decide whether he is sick or not (whether his orthopathy is intact, slightly disturbed, or seriously disrupted). The doctor should not be the one to suggest to him (or to inform him) that he is suffering from a headache, body aches, nausea, fatigue, or whatever it might be; the individual should be able to judge this for himself. The quantitative data supplied by somatic, causal-analytic medicine frequently (though certainly not always) is quite unconnected with basic assertions of this kind, which provide us with information about individual orthopathy (rather than pathology). An individual may have a delayed heartbeat (i.e., delayed with respect to the statistical norm) or low blood pressure and feel perfectly well all the same (or perhaps all the more). A second individual may feel that he is at his best and most energetic when his heart rate is "abnormally" high; a third individual, with an extremely elevated white blood cell count—which Western medicine generally takes as a signal for immediate intervention—may feel perfectly capable of going about the business of life as usual; while a fourth person may be plagued with chronic fatigue symptoms even though his white blood cell count is ostensibly normal.

Analytic medicine that relies entirely on quantitative data and uses a set of relative, normal values as an absolute standard is obliged to interpret every significant deviation from these values as "abnormal" if not actually "pathological." And, of course, in cases where there are no apparent deviations from the quantitative norm, analytic medicine is deprived of a rational basis on which to proceed with therapy.

Example: Tachycardia

Let us take a moment to develop this point a little farther by examining an extremely common phenomenon like tachycardia—an accelerated pulse rate, or a "pounding heart." In this case we are not talking about the kind of accelerated heart rate that normally follows a brief period of exertion and then subsides after a certain interval, of its own accord. There are countless varieties of tachycardia that must be regarded as "pathological," however—and anyone who experiences them definitely feels there is something wrong. Tachycardia is associated, for example, with a number of infectious febrile diseases, and when the disease itself is completely cured—as befits the special genius of Western medicine— then the patient's heart rate returns to normal, and we would be justified in describing this as causal therapy. However, tachycardia much more frequently occurs spontaneously, not in response to stress or any other perceptible stimulus, even sometimes when the individual is asleep or at rest. In many of these cases the quantitative methods employed in Western medicine are unable to discover any other significant deviation from recognized normal values. This does leave the alternative of directly stimulating by chemical means the nerves that regulate the activity of the heart muscle, but this is symptomatic rather than causal therapy—which completely begs the question of what effects this therapy is likely to have on the rest of the patient's body.

Naturally, Chinese medicine draws this same distinction between

152   normal and pathological forms of tachycardia. In either case, an accelerated pulse rate is regarded as a symptom, the product of some dynamic agency that must be precisely identified. A rapid pulse is primarily associated with *calor* (which literally means "heat," and is one of the eight leading diagnostic criteria referred to earlier and that we shall be examining shortly in some detail). It remains to be seen, however, whether this is merely an isolated symptom of *calor* or whether the majority of the other observable symptoms—or all of them without exception—also point in this direction. In the case of an acute infectious disease, the latter is most probably the case and the appropriate therapy is relatively straightforward. In the case of a chronic illness, there will be at most a few other clear-cut symptoms of *calor* accompanied by a vast profusion of additional symptoms that involve only the activities of certain function circles or that can be observed only at certain times of day. This is where the task of differential diagnosis begins—in precisely and unambiguously identifying all of these small-scale and often very subtle deviations from orthopathy.

Even in the case of a complicated diagnosis like this (assuming it is individual-specific and unqualifiedly positive), a specific therapy (aimed at a particular goal) and a definite prognosis may be possible, especially since, no matter what therapeutic methods are employed, they can be continuously monitored by the same diagnostic procedures and thus periodically reevaluated in detail and appropriately modified where necessary. For example, a case of intermittent but more or less chronic tachycardia—which would be explained away with such vague and unhelpful phrases as "congenital defect" and "emotional stress" by the average Western physician—might elicit a highly specific and unequivocal Chinese diagnosis, such as *inanitas yin orbis venalis* (depletion of constructive energy in the function circle of the kidneys) accompanied by a partial depletion of active energy in the circle of the liver and a total deficiency of constructive energy in the circle of the heart. (And in such a case one would also expect to have this diagnosis confirmed by the presence of a number of other symptoms besides the accelerated pulse rate, including sleep disorders, forgetfulness, frequent slips of the tongue, obsessiveness or *idées fixes,* and an unstable emotional life. A specific therapy that is precisely administered and that treats the underlying disorder rather than merely the symptoms will be able to restore orthopathy for all vital functions and to dispose of these additional symptoms as well as the tachycardia.)

THE PULSE DIAGNOSTIC

The Chinese doctor is not concerned with quantitative data, but because he is concerned with the overall pattern of relationships among all observable data, his diagnosis is often much more precise, more differentiated, and less ambiguous than a Western-style diagnosis would be. When a Western doctor takes a patient's pulse, for instance, all that he is interested in, apart from the pulse rate itself, is its relative strength or weakness, from which he may be able to draw certain inferences about the state of the patient's heart and circulatory system. Consequently it does not make any difference whether he feels the pulse on the patient's left wrist or his right, but in Chinese medicine this distinction is very important indeed in terms of the overall theoretical context in which all empirical data are evaluated. (More specifically, the characteristics of the left-hand pulse provide certain information about the function circles of the heart, the liver, the kidneys, the small intestine, the gall bladder, and the bladder; the right-hand pulse provides information about the circles of the lungs, spleen, large intestine, stomach, and the tricalorium.)

A second important distinction involves the relative location of the pulse point on the wrist—adjacent to the curved line on the palm that defines the ball of the thumb as it intersects with the wrist (called the "fishbelly boundary" by the Chinese). There are three pulse points, each about a finger's breadth across, on each hand, called *cun* ("thumb," *pollex*), *guan* ("straits" or "mountain pass," *clusa*), and *chi* ("foot," *pes*). Each pulse point (*situs*) corresponds to a pair of function circles, or, according to a different interpretation, the two *pollex* points (*pulsus pollicares*), one on each hand, correspond to the upper body (from the head to the chest), the *pulsus clusales* correspond to the midsection (from the chest to the navel), and the *pulsus pedales* to the lower body.

LABORATORY MEDICINE

In Western medicine, a positive diagnostic finding is actually an assertion about certain somatic activity *that has already concluded in the past.* The observation that a patient has a highly elevated white blood cell count (on which a Western doctor might base a diagnosis of leukemia) thus relies on somatic evidence of a cumulative functional disorder that has persisted over a relatively long period of time. The analysis of tissue samples also provides Western doctors with inferential evidence about *past* dysfunctions—e.g., analysis of liver tissue might suggest that a

154 patient has suffered from alcoholism or some other nutritional deficiency. Naturally, Western doctors have learned from their collective medical experience to draw certain conclusions from the evidence of these past perturbations about their patients' present and future states of being, but their "conclusions" are essentially just hypotheses or suppositions that have a greater or lesser probability of coming true. They are inherently less rigorous—less securely based on the evidence, in other words—than those assertions that are based on observable evidence of current functional activity (i.e., that are going on at this very moment). This distinction becomes all the more apparent in the case of various lab tests in which blood, urine, or tissue samples are analyzed at some remove, to put it mildly, from their original context. (In Europe this may even involve a transatlantic flight and a distance of several thousand miles, since the tests to detect certain prenatal metabolic disorders can be performed only at specially equipped laboratories in America.)

This point may require some clarification, however. Though it is true that assertions about present or future functional activity that are based on measurements of past functional activity are always, by definition, purely hypothetical, it is also true (as the record of every causal-analytical science has amply demonstrated) that such assertions may be successfully invoked to evaluate or to predict present or future functional activity in those cases where the factor we referred to earlier as "the homogeneity of the substrate" is relatively high (where the tissue or other substance that is involved in this activity is most nearly homogeneous in composition). In such a case, assertions about past functional activity will most probably hold true for the present and future as well, but of course as this homogeneity decreases, then the gap between hypothesis and reality grows wider. And, as we have already mentioned, the tacit assumption of Western medicine that such hypotheses will remain valid for a limited time in the future does in fact hold true in a great many but by no means all cases. It does not hold true for functional disorders that produce no *somatic* symptoms—pains of various kinds, diminished physical capacity, exhaustion or "nervous prostration," gradual loss of visual acuity (or of hearing, etc.). Only Chinese medicine is able to make scientifically precise assertions about cases of this kind.

This also implies that because the Western doctor is relying primarily on the evidence of past events, in the case of some disorders he does not really know what is going on until it is much too late. But a heart attack, a gastric ulcer, a gallstone attack, or an inflamed appendix is not a "spontaneous" infirmity that appears full-blown out of nowhere in a

matter of seconds; all of these result from severely protracted disruptions
of certain vital functions.

With Chinese medicine, the situation is quite different. The doctor does not collect quantitative data and thus may have no idea of what a patient was suffering from the day before or half an hour earlier. But the Chinese doctor is just as aware of his patient's current distress as the patient is himself; this presupposes that the Chinese doctor has access to certain diagnostic techniques that are just as precise and reliable as the Western doctor's quantitative measurements. We have already had a few words of introduction to the pulse diagnostic, the most important of these techniques, but so far we have said very little about the kind of qualitative assertions that comprise a Chinese diagnosis and what they actually consist of.

QUALITATIVE ASSERTIONS AND NORMATIVE CONVENTIONS

We would like to approach this subject somewhat indirectly by turning to the world of competitive sports to provide a good example of what we mean by "qualitative" assertions. What is there to say about a hundred-meter run, a javelin throw, or a soccer game apart from the quantitative outcome—time, distance, number of goals scored—particularly while the game or the event is still in progress? One might say, for example, that a particular runner is in remarkably good form, that the javelin is going up in a steep or shallow trajectory, or that the goalie has just successfully blocked a penalty kick. Certainly the records of the performance and the relative standing of a team or an individual athlete are measured in terms of certain predetermined qualitative factors. However, it is the *qualitative* factors that make a sporting event worth watching in the first place, or even "one for the books" or "truly unforgettable" (like the last match of the World Cup Final at Bern in 1954). And—to pursue the analogy a little farther—if Western doctors might be likened to the officials, the linesmen, or the judges (who collect the quantitative data), then Chinese doctors would be more like the coaches and trainers (who pick up on the athletes' mistakes and work relentlessly with them in order to correct them). In short, they judge the athletes' performances qualitatively.

In a strictly medical context now, this means that a Chinese diagnosis not only identifies the dynamic characteristics of the function circles involved but also tries to determine the direction or the course that an illness is going to take. One question we would like to discuss is, How

156   can these qualitative assertions claim to be *precise* (in the absence of quantitative standards)? More specifically, are these assertions "intersubjectively verifiable"? (Scientific work is said to be "intersubjectively verifiable" if a colleague can achieve the same results or reach the same conclusions quite independently—without being aware of the first scientist's thought processes or trying to "read his mind," in other words.) For this to be possible, these two scientists would have to share certain fundamental assumptions, of the sort that all scientific communities, all scientists who subscribe to the same theories or work in the same discipline have in common; e.g., they would both have to agree how long a meter or a second is; quantitative normative conventions are based on actual physical measurements.

As we have seen, the fact that Chinese science is based on qualitative rather than quantitative norms does not imply that Chinese scientists lacked the technical wherewithal to make the necessary measurements; instead, the reasons for this are theoretical—epistemological, if you will. Motion, current, contemporaneous events, and functions are necessarily incapable of being measured in this way, even with the most delicate instruments, because they have no "edges," no definite boundaries. Any attempt to impose a quantitative standard on Chinese medicine is necessarily doomed to failure for this very reason. To ask a Chinese doctor to produce the quantitative data on which he has based his diagnosis is a little like asking a biologist who informs you that blackbirds are nesting in a particular linden tree what measurements he proposes to make to support this hypothesis. A biologist (or an orchardman or an ordinary gardener) can recognize an apple tree in the spring when it is just coming into bud, in the summer when it is in full bloom, in the fall when it is laden with fruit, and in the winter when all its leaves have fallen. He can recognize it in the young seedling that has just broken out of the ground or even in the stack of firewood piled up at his feet.

The quantitative approach is clearly not necessary or even applicable here, but a scientist still must have some way of explaining to his colleagues how he has arrived at an assertion of this kind. In other words, science must be able to explain itself—its principles must be able to be taught, its discoveries communicated, its conclusions replicated and verified—rationally and unambiguously (this is one of the things that differentiates a science from an art or a craft, that differentiates medical science, for example, from a strictly empirical folk medicine). And since Chinese medicine concerns itself largely with phenomena that are either so fleeting as to be almost instantaneous (human speech, for example) or are still far short of completion (such as a human life), we have already seen how the quantitative method would not be very helpful in addressing any of these tasks (since in order for something to be measured, it must have exact, well-defined limits or boundaries). Thus—and this should perhaps not come as too much of a surprise—the precision, verifiability, communicability, and all the other scientific pillars of Chinese medicine must necessarily rest on a qualitative foundation. In fact, all of these scientific prerequisites can be fulfilled by means of the same sort of qualitative criteria by which, as we have already seen, a Chinese doctor can discern an orderly and coherent pattern of correspondences against an incalculably complex phenomenal backdrop that involves an almost infinite number of external influences and internal energy exchanges. And, as we have seen, all of these "wild" experiential phenomena can be tamed by being assigned a *direction* or some other qualitative characteristic (which really comes to the same thing).

We have already encountered a few of these qualitative normal values, such as *yin* and *yang,* which are terms that are no less universally understood than such familiar pairs of qualitative criteria as *right* and *left* in ordinary life or *negative* and *positive* in the world of physics. But Chinese medicine also concerns itself with qualitative distinctions that are even subtler and finer than many of the quantitative values and gradations that are adopted by Western medicine in order to present their empirical findings as a well-ordered sequence of quantitative terms. Chinese medicine thus possesses an even more variegated palette of qualitative values (though not sufficiently numerous as to become muddy or incoherent)—these are also employed, though in a somewhat different way, in acu-moxa-therapy and in the prescription of traditional remedies. Like the meter, the erg, or the second, these qualitative norms provide a common basis of communication and understanding for a scientific community. Apart from the cycle of the five transformation phases we have already encountered, they include the so-called *eight leading criteria* (*bagang*) and the *pathological agents* (*bingyin*), namely the six *climatic excesses* (*linyin*) and the *seven emotions* (*qi qing*). These are the most important criteria for unequivocal identification of a particular illness— for a diagnosis, in a word—and they will also enable us, eventually, to arrive at our own differential definition of the Chinese concept of illness or disease strictly according to the criteria of Chinese medicine. (So far all that we have really established in this respect is that Chinese doctors think of illness in terms of a continuous disruption of the operation of the function circles.)

Diagnostic Signs and Signals

THE eight leading criteria comprise four pairs of normative values of opposite polarity that provide a Chinese doctor with his first general (and generalizable) description of an individual patient's symptoms. We have already seen how *yin* and *yang* may be used as diagnostic indicators (corresponding to a hypothetical disruption of the flow of constructive or active energy, respectively); as *The Yellow Prince's Classic* puts it, "When *yin* and *yang* are in an anomalous relationship, then pathological disturbances will result." (Kidney stones, for example, are regarded as a *yin* symptom.)

The distinction between the "surface" (*biao, species*) and the "interior" (*li, intima*) provides us with a second pair of such criteria. A third, which we have already mentioned once or twice in passing, is the distinction between "heat" (*re, calor*) and "cold" (*han, algor*). Finally, there is the distinction between "exhaustion" (*xu, inanitas*) and "overabundance" (*shi, repletio*), which is a somewhat puzzling one at first, since *xu* refers to the depletion of certain kinds of energy (and thus a departure from orthopathy) and *shi* refers to the overabundance of other kinds of energy, which also results in a heteropathy.

YIN *AND* YANG *AS DIAGNOSTIC INDICATORS*

When we speak of a *yin* (constructive) symptom or disorder, this can mean either of two things. First, the material or physical aspect of the individual is in some way damaged, diminished, decaying, or disintegrating, or even (in part) destroyed. Second (and quite a different thing), the dynamic aspect of the individual has reached a "constructive" impasse of some sort—described variously as hardening or stiffening, becoming fixed or rigid, or in general "slowing down" or losing its dynamic force through some other kind of transformation. This first case would be designated as an "exhaustion of constructive potential"

160   (*inanitas yin*), the second as "constructive overabundance" (*repletio yin*), which might be imagined as an accumulation of divisive, deviant, or, in a word, heteropathic (*xie*) functions or quantities of energy. In the first case this involves a depletion or diminution of the kind of orthopathic constructive energy that provides the individual with the qualities of firmness and steadiness (for example, the so-called wasting or consumptive diseases). The second case involves the appearance of abnormal growths of tissue (*neoplasms,* as they are called in Western medicine) that act as a hindrance to bodily movement. In both cases, however, many of the same *yin* symptoms may present themselves, beginning with a dirty-white to greenish-white complexion. The patient is typically fatigued and reluctant to move, remains in a cramped or contorted position, or simply stays in bed. He feels weak and listless. The blade of the tongue is pale, swollen, and tender; the coating of the tongue is moist, smooth, and slippery. The patient's breathing is heavy and labored, and he may sometimes have difficulty speaking. His voice is weak and faint. His appetite for food and drink will be impaired, especially the former; he may prefer hot drinks, if anything. The urine is clear; the stool smells of fish or meat. The skin (especially on the arms and legs) is cold. At times the patient may experience abdominal pains that respond favorably to pressure (which accounts for the characteristic cramped or crouching posture). The pulse is (among other things) always very weak.

In a diagnostic context, *yang* also refers to two very different conditions. In the first case, there has been a repletion of the orthopathic active energy that supplies the dynamic aspect—the motive force, in other words, of the individual's ordinary life in the world. In the second case, certain processes that are associated with such *yang* qualities as expansion, dispersion, heat, and motion have had a heteropathic effect (i.e., the net result of all their operations has been a deviation from the functional optimum of the system). The symptoms of this first group are scarcely to be distinguished from those of the *yin* disorders mentioned earlier, but the symptoms of the second group are quite distinctive. The patient's complexion is very ruddy (or merely red in patches). The lips are dry and occasionally cracked. The blade of the tongue ranges from deep red to scarlet in color, the coating from yellow to yellowish-white (the color of quicklime). In serious cases, the surface of the tongue may even be dry and cracked, occasionally almost black in color and covered with warty excrescences. The patient is restless and constantly feels the urge to be in motion. His voice is strong and shrill, and he tends to curse and to cry out loud. The patient is garrulous and often confused in his speech. His breathing is loud and comes in gasps, sometimes accompanied by a kind of croupy cough. Since an overabundance of *yang* energy tends to dissipate the body's natural fluids, a patient with *yang* symptoms will often complain of a dry mouth and an excessive thirst. (He will also constantly feel hot and ask to be cooled off in some way.) Urine is reduced in volume and dark in color. The patient will be feverish, or he may experience unpleasant burning sensations. The pulse will probably be strong.

The classic texts describe the characteristic symptoms in contrasting pairs. Thus, *The Yellow Prince's Classic:* "If an *inanitas yang* predominates, the patient will feel cold on the outside; if *inanitas yin,* the patient will be aware of an inner heat. If *yang* is present in great abundance, the patient will feel warm on the outside; if *yin* is present in great abundance, he will feel cold on the outside."[2] Similarly, from elsewhere in the same source: "If active energy (*yangqi*) is overabundant, the body will be warm without sweat; if constructive energy is overabundant, there will be sweat without warmth."[3] A later work titled the *Shanghan Zabinglun* ("Treatise on *Algor*-Induced Disorders") states that "heat [fever] with shivering comes from [a misdirection of] the active principle; shivering without heat comes from [a misdirection of] the constructive principle."[4]

In practice, however, a patient is unlikely to exhibit symptoms of exclusively one kind or the other (and this holds true for the other three pairs of leading criteria as well). It is possible for a patient to present only *yin* (or *yang*) symptoms, of course, but this is only one possibility out of a very great many and is much more the exception than the rule. Generally symptoms belonging to these two categories tend to occur simultaneously and to shade off into one another on a continuum.

But at this point one might raise the objection that if certain diseases were always accompanied by a characteristic package of externally visible (or otherwise immediately verifiable) symptoms, then certainly this fact could not have remained entirely hidden from Western doctors as well, at least in the case of the simpler and more prevalent illnesses like the flu (certain forms of viral infection, in other words). But whether or not someone gets the flu depends on other things besides the virus's having gotten into his body somehow. This is, as the philosophers like to put it, a necessary but not a sufficient cause. Other factors might also be involved—the state of his immunological defenses (to use Western terminology), emotional stress, the weakening of the entire organism by a previous illness, and so forth. In Chinese medicine each of these factors would be duly considered as deviations from or disruptions of ortho-

162   pathy, and in each case would result in a different diagnosis. If a different clinical image of the underlying disorder emerges in each case, and if each of these patients later does come down with influenza or Queensland fever or some other infectious disease, then (from the standpoint of Chinese diagnosis) it is entirely a matter of chance which particular virus or bacteria they might have happened to come into contact with. A Western diagnosis of "flu" or "grippe" would thus be regarded as a generic term for a group of very similar but still differentiable illnesses that exhibit different symptoms—the difference here being all the more pronounced, since the identification of the "pathogen" (which is the entire basis, after all, of Western scientific medicine) plays an entirely subordinate role in Chinese medicine.

SPECIES *AND* INTIMA

These criteria can give the doctor additional information about the gravity of an illness, depending on whether it "takes hold" in the "exterior" of the body (closer to the surface) or the "interior." The original Chinese terms *biao* ("outside") and *li* ("inside") originally referred to the outside and the inside, or the lining, of a garment, and the ways in which these terms have been used in the medical literature are not always consistent. In the early texts (e.g., *The Yellow Prince's Classic*) *li* and *biao* were associated with the inner and outer function circles, respectively (for which we have also used the terms *intima* and *species*). Later, due to the influence of a very flexible conception of pathology, *biao* (*species*) came to describe the external or superficial regions of the body (the hair, skin, and the arterial pathways). *Li* thus came to refer to *both* the storage and the passage circles as well as the *paraorbes* (supplementary function circles) of the bones and the marrow.

"External" illnesses, at any rate, are characterized by fever and shivering, headaches, painfully sensitive areas on the torso and the limbs (whose boundaries can be precisely defined), a stopped-up nose, and a thin, whitish coating on the tongue. Symptoms of "internal" illnesses include high fever, restlessness, thirst, thoracic or abdominal pains, constipation, or diarrhea. The volume of urine is diminished; its color is described as reddish. The coating of the tongue is yellow or grayish-black. (We should also mention in passing that both *intima* and *species* disorders are associated with certain distinctive pulse patterns.)

It seems safe to conclude from this that "superficial" (*species*) illnesses are more or less that—less serious, not life-threatening, perhaps about to disappear of their own accord. Serious, deep-seated, stubborn, persistent, or chronic illnesses are always classified as *intima,* and since certain illnesses develop from *species* to *intima,* Chinese medicine also recognizes the symptoms that mark this transition.

ALGOR *AND* CALOR

The Chinese words *han* and *re* literally mean "cold" and "heat"; in this case we feel it is particularly appropriate to use the Latin equivalents *algor* and *calor,* if only to serve as a reminder that these terms are not merely descriptive, that they actually represent highly abstract principles of classification that can be applied to a great many phenomena that could not be described as being hot or cold in any literal sense. Thus a yellow coating on the tongue or a very agitated manner of speaking are classified as *calor* symptoms (to choose just two examples among many), whereas an exceptionally slick coating on the tongue and an extreme reluctance to say anything are classified as *algor* symptoms. Admittedly febrile symptoms are classified as *calor,* for the most part, and many that are associated with chills are classified as *algor,* but numerically these are not very significant in a much broader diagnostic context.

Besides being quiet to the point of taciturnity, a patient with *algor* symptoms also requires a great deal of rest; he lies in bed with his knees drawn up toward his chest. His eyes will appear to be clear and moist (though the patient may prefer to keep them closed). His complexion is pale, perhaps verging on greenish-white. The lips and the fingernail crescents tend to be bluish-violet; the tongue is colorless to pale pink, with a whitish coating or without any coating at all. The patient may experience violent retching, and he may bring up a thin, clear, or whitish liquid. The urine is clear and abundant, but there may be a tendency toward diarrhea. The patient will drink very little but will continue to salivate copiously. Occasionally he will have a craving for warm foods. His hands and feet will be cold.

A composite picture of the typical *calor* symptoms gives us a patient who is red-faced, talkative, and rather loud (as opposed to pale, taciturn, and quiet). The patient will lie flat on his back in bed and is inclined to be restless. The lips are dry and cracked (or puffy) and red in color; the crescents of the fingernails range in color from red to violet. The blade of the tongue will appear to be hard, leathery, and furrowed; the coating is thick and dry, sometimes prickly to the touch, and ranges in color from yellow to black. The patient may vomit large quantities of a viscous yellowish fluid; he may also be suffering from constipation, and his urine will be sparse and dark yellow to reddish in color. He will continually

164   crave cold drinks, and his mouth will always be dry. His limbs will feel warm to the touch.

Once again, it is important to bear in mind that these are the typical symptoms of *algor* and *calor* but that a patient who only exhibited symptoms of one kind or the other would hardly be typical at all. (Surely each of us can recall certain occasions when we have been laid up in bed with a raging fever and ice-cold feet.) To further complicate the picture, there are certain atypical symptoms, referred to collectively as "false *algor*" and "false *calor*," that can mislead an inexperienced practitioner into making an incorrect diagnosis and administering an inappropriate treatment, which can' result in serious complications of the original illness.[5] As for what the appropriate therapy might consist of, we shall have to content ourselves for the moment by repeating a typically sententious observation from *The Yellow Prince's Classic:* "*Algor* must be warmed up and *calor* must be cooled off."

INANITAS *AND* REPLETIO

As we have seen, these two principles generally operate in tandem with *yin* and *yang* as diagnostic criteria. To recapitulate briefly, Chinese medicine makes an important distinction between disorders that are caused by an insufficiency or a depletion of orthopathic energy (*inanitas*) on the one hand (the term literally means "emptiness" or "exhaustion") and by an overabundance of heteropathic energy (*repletio*)—i.e., energy whose normal flow has somehow been blocked or misdirected and thus has given rise to a disruption of the normal dynamic equilibrium. It is worth noting that these two terms do not refer to two different states of the same reservoir of energy—"approaching empty" and "overflowing," or the like—since *inanitas* refers to a drop in the level of the patient's "physiological" energy reserves, whereas *repletio* refers to an abnormal accumulation of energy that is inaccessible to or isolated from the individual's normal reserves of energy.

As the name itself suggests, the appropriate therapy for *inanitas* would involve whatever measures are necessary to supplement or help to replenish or mobilize the individual's remaining reserves of energy. *Repletio* would seem to require more vigorous intervention to disperse or drain off or neutralize the excess energy. It also seems clear enough that except in the case of a highly acute disorder where the patient's life is threatened, the restoration of orthopathy will generally take precedence over a more direct assault on the heteropathy. The primary goal of the treatment, after all, is to restore the patient to his normal state of

health—*restitutio ad integrum* is the equivalent phrase in classical
Western medicine—and not simply to root out and destroy the heteropathy. The use of such words as "disperse," "drain off," and "neutralize"
correctly implies that this process, even if conducted on a modest and
unpretentious scale, also puts a strain on the patient's already depleted
resources. (In the case of a sufficiently massive heteropathy that has
already taken on material form [neoplasia], this may even involve
permanent injury to the patient.) This principle is primarily of importance in cases where symptoms of both *inanitas* and *repletio* are present,
of course, so that treatment would primarily be directed at the former.

We have already mentioned that every individual is thought to
contain two different forms of "individual-specific" energy (i.e., energy
whose precise nature or characteristics are different in each individual
case). The active form of energy is called *qi,* the constructive form *xue,*
and both may become depleted or anomalously overabundant in the
ways we have been discussing. This provides us with four somewhat
more precise diagnostic criteria to work with: *inanitas qi, repletio qi,
inanitas xue,* and *repletio xue.* (To avoid inflicting both *inanitas* and
repletio on the reader, however, we shall present only an abbreviated list
of symptoms for these first two categories, solely for purposes of
comparison.)

Inanitas qi symptoms, grouped by the relevant functional regions,
might include shortness of breath or even asthma; a soft, breathless voice,
and spontaneous outbreaks of sweating; abdominal pains that respond
favorably to pressure; loss of appetite accompanied by dyspepsia and
diarrhea, and perhaps abdominal swelling as well. The hands and feet
may feel cold and weak, perhaps even numb. Additional symptoms may
include a strained, husky voice (the patient may even have difficulty
speaking), saliva dribbling out of the mouth, alternate dilation and
contraction of the pupils, and twitching of the eyelids and the hands or
limbs; tachycardia, irregular breathing, ringing in the ears (tinnitus),
dizziness, and temporary loss of hearing (as the result of fatigue or
exhaustion).

Repletio qi symptoms may include bronchial congestion (so that the
patient characteristically tends to keep his chest braced in the "exhale"
position) accompanied by breathing problems that may become unbear-
able when the patient is lying down. The stomach rumbles, and he will
be troubled with belching (accompanied by a sour or unpleasant smell).
He may have the sensation of choking or constant nausea, and in
extreme cases this may prevent him from eating anything or keeping

166   anything down. Additional symptoms include a fever that periodically rises and falls, stool flecked with red or white patches, and confused and irrational speech.

TAXONOMIC PIGEONHOLES AND DIAGNOSTIC CRITERIA

We could continue this recital almost indefinitely, but the real point we are trying to make is that with these eight leading criteria Chinese medical theory provides the doctor with a systematic framework for the evaluation of a vast multiplicity of diagnostic signs and symptoms. This method of classifying symptoms by means of these qualitative conventions is both precise and flexible enough (even in describing their various relationships with one another) that the doctor need not attach too much importance to any individual symptom, which, if it is ambiguous or ill-defined, can simply be disregarded. A Chinese doctor could never bring himself to admit that an illness could not somehow betray its presence by any number of symptoms, though it is very much in keeping with the inductive-synthetic character of Chinese medicine that such individual details are not permitted to distract one's attention from the overall image of the patient's illness that emerges from this schematic representation of his symptoms.

In practical terms this also means that when a Chinese doctor encounters certain symptoms that he believes (based on his own practical experience and rational judgment) are not worth categorizing as significant deviations from the patient's functional optimum, then he will make no attempt to incorporate them into this diagnostic framework. If the patient's lips, let us say, are neither bright red nor abnormally pale, then the question of what color they actually are (and what qualitative criterion this might be associated with) is utterly moot. If the patient's pulse at a particular *situs* is neither especially rapid nor sluggish, then nothing more needs to be said about it.

Conversely, let us suppose that the patient's face is a bright, flaming red (so much so that even a layman would be struck by it). This is a critical symptom that should be identified by means of one of the leading criteria (perhaps *yang, calor,* or *repletio*). This will prove useful if the remaining symptoms, though well defined in themselves, would appear to the layman or to the patient himself to be contradictory or inconsistent (as is frequently the case with serious or chronic disorders). The patient may be sweating and shivering simultaneously; he may have a high temperature, even a fever, and still refuse to drink anything; or he may have a craving for cold drinks even though he finds them nauseating as soon as he has gotten them down. There are many other possible diagnostic paradoxes of this kind, and these provide the real test of a mature, rational system of diagnosis; these are also the sort of cases, of course, that test whether the doctor's acquaintance with this great legacy of diagnostic expertise is profound or merely superficial.

Naturally, one might object that, e.g., any one of the individual *calor* or *repletio* symptoms we mentioned in the previous section *in and of itself* is imprecisely described or simply of dubious diagnostic value (the pitch and timbre of the patient's voice, perhaps). But the fact is that in Chinese medicine symptoms are never evaluated in and of themselves but rather as elements in a comprehensive and synchronistic pattern of diagnostic indicators. The empirical methods employed by Chinese doctors are essentially no different from those of their Western counterparts, but they do evaluate their empirical observations from a very different perspective, and they have learned to take certain factors into account that Western doctors would tend to disregard. This unique vantage point is provided by the eight "leading criteria"—criteria for assigning a precise qualitative direction to each of these phenomena—which allow the Chinese doctor to classify and thus to discriminate between physiological and pathological processes that might otherwise appear to be identical. To view the achievements (to say nothing of the potential) of Chinese medicine in the proper context, we must bear in mind that hundreds of physiological functions that, judging by Western standards, would appear to be quite unrelated have been arranged into a coherent system involving only five (or six) pairs of complementary function circles by means of the science of orbisiconography. This in turn permits hundreds of different pathological symptoms to be rationally classified for diagnostic purposes by assigning them to the appropriate function circles. Chinese medical theory did not develop as a purely speculative exercise or in isolation from the concerns of practical medicine but rather was built up gradually and organically as an expandable array of taxonomic compartments—pigeonholes, if you will—for the sorting of empirical data and has since developed into a true medical science of remarkable consistency and clinical efficiency.

THE PATHOLOGICAL AGENTS

Although the eight leading criteria provide Chinese medicine with a relatively fine-meshed technique of differential diagnosis, the primary purpose of diagnosis, after all, is not just to classify symptoms but rather

168   to identify the more basic, underlying factors associated with an illness, which in Chinese medicine are called "pathological agents" (*yin* or *bingyin*). The main difference between the concept of a "pathological agent" in the Chinese inductive-synthetic system and what we would ordinarily call a "cause" in the Western causal-analytic system is that a pathological agent is thought to exist simultaneously with its effects rather than preceding them in time. This surely corresponds with experience in certain respects, and those of us who are susceptible to such things know that they are likely to keep getting headaches just as long as a warm, steady wind keeps blowing out of the south (whether they happen to call it the *Föhn,* the *antan,* or the Santa Ana), just as we all know that we are likely to keep on shivering just as long as we keep standing in the cold or that the risk of getting a sunburn immediately drops to nil as soon as we step into the shade.

To practitioners of Western medicine, and others, this may seem to be merely a trivial or a pedantic distinction. It is perfectly obvious that both Chinese and Western doctors are predominantly concerned with the treatment of disorders that have already outlasted the immediate effects of the agency that brought them into being. (In other words, a potential sunburn might be prevented by stepping under a tree, but an actual, preexisting sunburn, to say nothing of sunstroke, could not be so easily disposed of.) But this would be evading the real issue as well, since from the Chinese perspective, as we have already learned, a disorder of any kind can be reliably identified only as it exists at the present moment. In answer to the objection that a sunburn makes its presence known and felt only some time after the initial exposure, a Chinese-style diagnosis would be able to detect certain striking departures from orthopathy almost as soon as the first ultraviolet rays had struck the skin of the prospective patient (who, of course, regards the experience as a rather pleasant one). A Western physician might have to wait for some time before he could detect the first somatic evidence (perhaps a measurable hyperemia of the skin, a progressive disturbance of the dermis and the epidermis or of the circulatory system in general).

Still, Chinese medicine clearly has to come to terms with the fact that certain disruptions of orthopathy may persist for hours, days, or years after the initial disruptive impulse has dissipated. This is accounted for by postulating the existence of a condition we have been referring to as heteropathy (*xie,* "crookedness"), which is defined not only as a departure from orthopathy but also, more specifically, as a quantity of energy that has been detached or diverted from (and thus may be acting in opposition to) the body's normal energy reserves. We will have occasion to refer back to this second definition in our discussion of the pathological agents and the characteristic disorders they give rise to.

For example, a pathological agent may be thought to aggravate a preexisting energy deficiency and thus to induce a number of heteropathies, to the detriment of the dynamic equilibrium of the individual. If this disruption is not too severe, the imbalance may be corrected and the heteropathy "absorbed"; otherwise it may simply persist in more or less its initial state, or it may continue to drain off physiological energy at an ever-increasing rate. At first this final turn of events would be evidenced by *repletio* symptoms in the area that had been isolated by the heteropathy and *inanitas* symptoms in the complementary functional region. If the initial attempts at treatment were to prove unsuccessful but if subsequent therapy was much too rigorous (and thus put too much of a strain on the patient), the original heteropathy would be dispersed only at the cost of a further disruption of orthopathy (but this time in the direction of *inanitas*). This, of course, would leave the patient extremely vulnerable to the further depredations of pathological agents in the near future.

In a section of *The Yellow Prince's Classic* that bears the imposing title "Commentary on the Words of Truth from the Golden Shrine," the Yellow Prince asks his mentor, "Since there are eight winds in the heavens, then why are there only five in the pathways of the body? What have you to say to that?" The Count of Qi replies, "The eight winds give rise to heteropathies, and it is these that become the winds of the arterial pathways. If they invade the five storage circles, then the heteropathies thus engendered will give rise in turn to sicknesses."[6] From a nontraditional perspective, perhaps the Count's answer might be taken to imply that such things are largely matters of descriptive convention and thus not to be taken too literally. The "sicknesses" that the count is referring to are very serious alterations in the direction of the interior function circles, but since illnesses are thought to take hold originally in the outer regions of the body, where the arterial pathways are located, the pathological agents responsible for these disorders are called the "five winds of the pathways." Identifying these pathological agents with the "winds of heaven" also implies quite clearly that certain heteropathies are more likely to manifest themselves at certain seasons of the year and that the risk of contracting an illness of this kind is greater at certain times than at others.

The winds of the pathways are only one of the six so-called climatic

170   excesses, which in turn are one of three groups of pathological agents recognized by Chinese medicine. As before, since the Chinese names for these phenomena often prove to be merely distracting rather than illuminating in a discussion of their precise use in Chinese medicine, we shall refer to them by their Latin equivalents. Thus the six climatic excesses include *ventus* (*feng,* "wind"), *algor* ("cold," though here the term refers to the external temperature rather than the body temperature), *aestus* ("oppressive summer heat"), *humor* ("dampness, moisture"), *ariditas* ("drought, dryness"), and *ardor* ("dry, fiery heat"). Next comes a second group of internal influences on individual orthopathy, the "seven emotions" (*qi qing*), consisting of *voluptas* ("desire"), *ira* ("anger"), *sollicitudo* ("worry"), *cogitatio* ("reflection"), *maeror* ("sorrow"), *timor* ("fear"), and *pavor* ("terror"). In addition, there are three "neutral" agents (i.e., neither internal nor external): poor nutrition, overexertion, and sexual excess.

As theoretical concepts, the pathological agents are useful in themselves as an additional qualitative index for the evaluation of empirical data as an aid to differential diagnosis. They also play a pivotal role in coordinating theoretical systems like orbisiconography and the theory of the transformation phases with their practical diagnostic applications. In this respect, it is important to note that in practice the heteropathies induced by the pathological agents are also referred to by the names listed above, so that a Chinese doctor might refer to a *ventus* (or rather *feng*) heteropathy or simply *ventus,* meaning the same thing in each case—since illnesses are likely to outlast the effects of the pathological agents responsible (which indeed is why the concept is both theoretically useful and necessary in the first place). In the following discussion it will also be helpful to bear in mind the basic axiom of orbisiconography, that all external influences on a function circle can be beneficial in the appropriate amount or intensity, and only when this optimum is exceeded will they become harmful.

THE SIX CLIMATIC EXCESSES

The Overstraining Factor: Ventus

The principal symptoms of a superficial *ventus* heteropathy (*ventus speciei*) include fever accompanied by shivering and chills, headaches, and neck pains. The patient is disoriented, has a slight cough, and speaks in a husky voice. His nose may be stuffed up as well, and his eyes may frequently fill up with tears. The coating on the tongue is thin and uniform. The function circle of the liver (and its complement, the circle of the gall bladder) are especially vulnerable to heteropathies of this kind, and patients who are suffering from disorders of these circles are advised in the *Suwen* to "take care to avoid these winds." In fact, the "winds of the body" and the other climatic excesses may result in energy imbalances in any of the function circles (and, of course, in their complements at the same time).

The symptoms of a more advanced heteropathy that has already penetrated into one of the function circles include shooting pains in the joints, restricted mobility and even partial paralysis of the facial muscles and the eyelids, attacks of dizziness or fainting spells, total loss of sensitivity in certain parts of the face, painful lumps or swellings beneath the skin, and skin eruptions, like German measles, that are accompanied by fever. *Ventus* is associated with the transformation phase of wood and is particularly likely to manifest itself in the spring. It is also unique among the six climatic excesses in that it has the potential of combining with any one of the others to produce a kind of composite disorder that is referred to as *algor venti, aestus venti,* or whatever the case might be.

The Crippling Factor: Algor

In practice, it is unlikely that the two separate concepts referred to as *algor* in Chinese medicine could ever be confused, since the referent of the *algor* we are currently considering is so much less specific, so much more inclusive and comprehensive than that of the diagnostic criterion *algor*. *Algor* is associated with the transformation phase of water (*yin* in *yin,* in other words), which naturally suggests an extreme constructive tendency and a pronounced deficiency of *yang* energy in the presence of an *algor* heteropathy. The circles of the bladder and the kidneys are particularly susceptible to these disorders (all the more so during the winter months).

Superficial symptoms of *algor* include fever accompanied by shivering and gooseflesh (rather than sweating), and pains in the head, neck, and back as far down as the lumbar region and perhaps elsewhere as well. An *algor* heteropathy in the arterial pathways results in muscle cramps and aching joints; the hands and feet will be tinged with a purplish-red color. If the *algor* penetrates into the function circles themselves, the patient will be troubled with abdominal pains and various internal rumblings, followed by vomiting or diarrhea. The blade of the tongue will be pale and will eventually acquire a white coating. "If the sickness prevails in the circle of the kidneys," warns *The Yellow Prince's Classic,* "then the

172   patient should beware of piping-hot food and clothing that has been warmed up for him on the stove." *Algor* heteropathies may be treated by the cautious application of "cool" remedies (this is a qualitative conventional term that we will encounter again in a subsequent chapter).

The Overtaxing Factor: Aestus

Aestus is associated with the transformation phase of fire and is particularly likely to affect two complementary pairs of function circles: the circles of the heart and the small intestine and the circles of the pericardium and the tricalorium. The initial symptoms are essentially those of mild "heat exhaustion" or "heat prostration," resembling fever symptoms accompanied by apathy and debilitation, even a kind of torpor, and sudden outbreaks of sweating. The patient is often disoriented and short of breath; his face will take on a sallow, "dirty" color. The blade of the tongue is red with a thin yellow coating; the urine is reddish, and the urinary flow is constricted. Heatstroke is an extreme form of *aestus* heteropathy.

Very different symptoms are presented by a patient who has made an ill-advised attempt to remedy his discomfort by, e.g., plunging into ice-cold water—shivering and damp, clammy skin, perhaps followed by abdominal cramps, nausea, and diarrhea (which demonstrates the functional involvement of the circles of the heart and the small intestine, as well as their particular vulnerability to disorders of this kind). We have all certainly been warned about "cramps" and the other unpleasant consequences of going swimming at inopportune times; the Chinese explanation for this is that extreme cold (constructivity) blocks the natural circulation of active energy.

If *aestus* is accompanied by *humor* ("dampness"), then the initial symptoms will be similar to those just mentioned, but both the circles of the small and of the large intestines will be involved; in extreme cases, this may lead to serious illness, including dysentery and cholera. In a hot and humid climate, as typified by the dog days in August, malarialike symptoms may also be present, or even malaria itself.

The Dampening Factor: Humor

Humor heteropathies may result from wearing clothing that has been soaked with rain or sweat or from frequenting moist or humid premises, or even from overindulging in fruits that have a lot of juice. *Humor* is associated with the transformation phase of earth and thus with the function circles of the spleen and the stomach. The corresponding *sapor* is sweet, and an excess of sweet-tasting foods can deplete the active energy reserves of the circle of the spleen. *Humor* symptoms are further classified into two categories, *inferior* and *superior*. The former includes severe menstrual cramps accompanied by an abnormally thick menstrual discharge; the latter includes nasal congestion and stertorous breathing. Superficial (*humor externus*) symptoms include prostration or exhaustion; outbreaks of sweating (when the air temperature is not particularly warm); and painful, swollen joints. *Humor internus* symptoms include a feeling of pressure inside the chest and swelling in the lower abdominal region, often accompanied by vomiting and loss of appetite. Jaundice and diarrhea are also associated with *humor internus.*

The Sharpening, Hardening Factor: Ariditas
Ariditas corresponds to the transformation phase of metal and thus to the function circles of the lungs and large intestine. Partaking of food or drink that is too cold, or wearing inadequate clothing are thought to be conducive to heteropathies of this kind, which are also classified into two subcategories: "cold" (*ariditas frigula*) and "warm" (*ariditas temperate*). Symptoms of "cold" *ariditas* include chills and shivering that are not accompanied by sweating, as well as coughing, neck pain, nasal congestion, and mild headaches. The coating of the tongue is white and dry. "Warm" *ariditas* symptoms include fever and sweating, neck pains, abnormal thirst, frequent coughing spells, and chest pains. The patient may cough up blood or mucus, and the coating of the tongue is dry and yellowish.

Hyperactivity: Ardor
In serious cases, all of these first five heteropathies may develop into *ardor,* which is associated with a loss of fluid (and thus of the individual's constructive energy reserves). Like *aestus, ardor* corresponds to the transformation phase of fire and thus is identified with an excess of *yang* energy. Symptoms include a high fever, restlessness, red face and bloodshot eyes, neck pains, and abnormal thirst. The blade of the tongue is deep red in color, the coating a dirty yellow and covered with pimply excrescences. (We should also mention that in practice the doctor's finding of *ardor, ariditas,* etc., can be confirmed by feeling the patient's pulse.)

THE SEVEN EMOTIONS
You may recall from our discussion of orbisiconography that each of the five original storage circles corresponds to a particular psychic reaction

174   (*emotio*): anger (*ira,* circle of the liver), pleasure or desire (*voluptas,* circle of the heart), pensiveness or reflection (*cogitatio,* circle of the spleen), worry (*sollicitudo,* circle of the lungs), and fear (*timor,* circle of the kidneys). For our present purposes this list is amended to include two additional emotions: sorrow (*maeror*), which also affects the function circle of the lungs, and terror (*pavor*), which depletes the energy reserves of the circle of the heart. It should be made clear that ordinary emotions are not regarded as pathological agents in themselves; however, extreme or exaggerated accesses of emotion—regarded more or less as the internal equivalent of the six climatic excesses—are thought to have a pathological effect on their corresponding function circles and to evince their presence by means of characteristic symptoms, which in turn permit certain inferences to be drawn about the current dynamic state of the function circles.

The complete repression of one's emotions, or the absence of any emotional response to anything, is also regarded as an emotional extreme and thus as a potentially pathological condition. This should not be interpreted as a kind of prescientific pop psychology—"Keeping all your emotions bottled up inside you is bad for you" and the like—since it does in fact rest on a scientific basis. It seems clear how the doctor's findings with respect to *inanitas* and *repletio* could be correlated with the patient's emotional reactions to provide additional information about the direction (i.e., a tendency either toward energy "exhaustion" or "congestion") an illness was likely to take and the extent to which particular function circles were already involved.

However, this theoretical explanation is unlikely to meet the objections of Western observers who are unwilling to admit that phenomena of this kind could possibly be of diagnostic value. Nor are they likely to be appeased at this point by the explanation that no individual symptom, in and of itself, is of diagnostic value unless it can be examined in the overall context of all observable symptoms. To this a Western doctor might very reasonably reply that even if he knew all about the climatic and emotional excesses affecting the patient, knew that he had a headache and felt too weak to do much of anything, had taken the patient's pulse and looked at his tongue, he would have no idea what the cause of his illness was. And to this, in turn, a Chinese doctor would quite correctly reply that he was not concerned in the least with the *cause* of the patient's illness but with its actual nature and the course it was likely to take in the future. It is important to remember here that these psychic reactions or emotions are primarily of interest not because they provide any information of behavioral or psychological significance about the patient but because they assist the doctor in arriving at certain conclusions about the state of the patient's vital functions in a particular instance.

Unrestrained Emotion: Voluptas ("Pleasure")

Pleasure, the psychic reaction associated with the function circle of the heart, is regarded as a great stimulus to the imagination and to the individual's reserves of building energy and defensive energy. When the individual becomes excessively preoccupied with pleasure, however, the result is likely to be an *inanitas* of the circle of the heart, which leads in turn to a diminution of the binding force that "holds him together" as an individual personality. The energy of the circle of the heart is thought to be blocked or baffled by the energy of the circle of the kidneys, which can result in such symptoms as disorientation and confused, incoherent speech; lack of muscular coordination; and random, disorganized behavior.

Repressed Emotion: Ira ("Anger")

Frequent or violent displays of anger overtax the energy reserves of the circle of the liver and its complement, the circle of the gall bladder, whereas a *repletio* of the circle of the liver may provoke an angry emotional outburst for no apparent reason. (This reversible relationship is typical of all the function circles and their complementary emotions.) As you may recall, the form of energy stored in the circle of the liver is *xue,* individual-specific constructive energy. A *repletio* of the circle of the liver also has an indirect effect on its "neighbors," the circles of the heart and the kidneys—*neighbors* in this case meaning its immediate successor in the first sequence of transformation phases and its complement. External symptoms associated with *ira* include, not surprisingly, a bright red face and, in extreme cases, even unconsciousness or cerebral hemorrhage.

Restrained Emotion: Sollicitudo ("Worry")

Severe anxiety is thought to have its most pronounced effects on the complementary circles of the lungs and the small intestine, which in turn may produce such symptoms as shortness of breath and coughing up large quantities of phlegm, perhaps accompanied by a distended abdo-

176   men and severe diarrhea. In general, anxiety has the effect of disrupting
the rhythm of all the vital functions, which has a marked effect on the
equalizing and integrating functions exercised by the circle of the spleen
and thus on the dynamic interplay of the energies of all the function
circles. This may give rise to a number of other symptoms in addition to
the foregoing—namely, shallow breathing accompanied by coughing
and loss of appetite, perhaps followed by a general loss of muscle tone,
which is first apparent in the hands and feet.

Disciplined Emotion: Cogitatio ("Reflection")

The conventional image of the great philosopher who can't remember
what he had for breakfast is in perfect accord with the tenets of Chinese
medicine, which holds that excessive reflection (to the exclusion of all
other psychic reactions and preoccupations) leads not only to forgetfulness but to lassitude and debilitation as well. Excessive reflection (though
generally what is meant by this is not so much abstract thought or
rumination as excessive introspection or brooding) has a disruptive effect
on the function circle of the spleen and thus on the underlying rhythm
of all the circles, so that symptoms may include tachycardia, "night
sweats," and loss of appetite (to the point of serious weight loss and
malnutrition). As we have just learned, the "executive" activities of the
spleen are also affected by severe anxiety (*sollicitudo*), which acts directly
on its immediate successor in the first sequence of the transformation
phases, the circle of the lungs. Certainly these two states of mind—worry
or anxiety on the one hand and pensiveness and excessive introspection
on the other—are not unrelated, and the reciprocal relationship between
the corresponding disorders of these two neighboring function circles
may be seen as analogous to the way in which anxiety and morbid
introspection seem to exacerbate and to feed on each other.

Overwhelming Emotion: Maeror ("Sorrow")

Regarded—in functional terms, at least—as a kind of adjunct to
sollicitudo, "worry," *maeror* also affects the function circle of the lungs,
and (in accordance with the principle that under pathological conditions
the transformation phase of fire may be "subdued" by the transformation
phase of metal) the circle of the heart—which corresponds with the
transformation phase of fire—may also be affected sympathetically,
resulting in the depletion of the energy reserves of both these circles. A
pale and haggard face is the only physical symptom of this condition; the
patient will also appear to be listless and apathetic.

Captive Emotion: Timor ("Fright")

The kind of dull, nameless fear that so many men and women carry around with them has become characteristic of our society. Western man sometimes seems to be doing rather well, but still this vague feeling of dread has inexplicably become our constant companion in prosperity. In Chinese medicine, groundless or irrational fear is ordinarily regarded as the result of an *inanitas* of the function circle of the kidneys. (Remember that in practice this would remain merely a hypothesis or a supposition until confirmed diagnostically in the usual way.) And, of course, a powerful fright (whether irrational or otherwise) is likely to have a deleterious effect on this function circle; the circle of the heart, as the successor of the circle of the kidneys in the second (conquering) transformational sequence (corresponding to fire and water, respectively), may also be affected. Symptoms associated with *timor* include depression, indecision, restlessness, and paranoia (accompanied by an irrational urge to cover oneself up or to conceal oneself from view).

Overmastering Emotion: Pavor ("Terror")

Unreasoning panic or terror may also drastically deplete the normal energy reserves of the circle of the heart, so that those who are already suffering from this condition are advised to stay away from any situation in which they might receive an additional shock of this kind. The symptoms are similar to those associated with *voluptas,* which also directly affects the circle of the heart: restlessness and rapid breathing, confused and incoherent speech, purposeless and inconsistent behavior. (The similarity of symptoms should not pose problems for the diagnostician, since the patient himself can readily distinguish between the craving for pleasure and an irrational feeling of terror.)

NEUTRAL PATHOLOGICAL AGENTS

As mentioned earlier, there are three additional agents that do not quite fit into the foregoing schema:

Improper Diet

Naturally enough, all the symptoms attributed to poor nutrition in Chinese medicine would be regarded as digestive disorders in the West: belching accompanied by a sour or unpleasant smell, heartburn, throwing up undigested food, and a feeling like a lump of lead in one's stomach, as well as pains and swellings in the region around the stomach. Insofar

178   as the circle of the spleen may be adversely affected by poor nutrition, this may result in either diarrhea or constipation.

Physical Overexertion

This can result in a pathological depletion of the individual's reserves of constructive energy as well as other reserves of energy throughout the body. The symptoms are surely familiar enough to all of us—total exhaustion, breathlessness, the feeling that one is too tired to sleep, and, in more serious cases, spontaneous outbreaks of sweating accompanied by a burning sensation and tachycardia.

Sexual Excesses

As far as Chinese medicine is concerned, sexual activity can be defined as excessive, and thus pathological, when the energy reserves of the circle of the kidneys become severely depleted. (Sexual functions, as you may recall, are assigned to the circle of the kidneys in orbisiconography.) Symptoms of such an *inanitas* include sweaty or clammy palms and soles of the feet, a feeling of weakness in the legs and hips, as well as (for men) nocturnal emissions, premature ejaculation and other sexual dysfunctions, and even atrophy of the genital organs. Here again, the circle of the heart may also be affected indirectly by a severe enough *inanitas* of the circle of the kidneys, which may give rise to a number of additional symptoms—coughing up bloody sputum, a low-grade fever (which appears at the same time every day), "night sweats," and tachycardia.

SUMMARY

Thus far we have encountered all sixteen of the pathological agents recognized as such in Chinese medicine—though the necessity of discussing them one by one and in isolation from their total context has tended to impose a kind of Western analytic (though decidedly not causal) perspective on our discussion. It very seldom happens that an illness can be ascribed to a single pathological agent, so that a wide variety of these symptoms are likely to be present in any given case. Strictly from the standpoint of common sense, it seems obvious enough, for example, that the same individual might be suffering from the ill effects of his poor eating habits and overexertion at the same time, and the idea that one's emotional difficulties and the less satisfactory aspects of one's environment might enter into the picture as well should not seem too farfetched.

We have also discovered how the eight leading criteria, which occupy an even more central position in the battle order of Chinese diagnostic medicine, can provide the doctor with information about the extent to which an illness has progressed and its probable future course. However, we could hardly put too much emphasis on the fact that this ability to interpret accurately the multiplicity of diagnostic data that presents itself for the doctor's inspection can be acquired only with clinical experience (in addition to a thorough grounding in the theoretical principles involved). In the People's Republic today, for example, a four-year course of study is prescribed for students of traditional medicine, and in former times it was customary for a student to spend many years, perhaps even several decades in the service of his teacher (who, of course, was often his own father) to learn the traditions and the unwritten lore of his profession at first hand. There is simply a great deal more there than can be absorbed by even the most attentive student during a three-week course in Chinese medicine, especially in the midst of the fleshpots of Taipei or Hong Kong.

The point we are trying to make is not that Chinese medical theory is especially complex or difficult to learn (surely no more than any other scientific discipline) but that we believe it to be well worth the effort of learning it. It points the way to the intriguing prospect of a thoroughly systematized, strictly logical science of healing. With this fairly modest conceptual armory at one's disposal—the transformation phases and the three transformational sequences, the sister disciplines of sinarteriology and orbisiconography, the eight leading diagnostic criteria, and the sixteen pathological agents we have just discussed—it should be possible to identify and systematize the virtually infinite variety of individual illnesses by means of a process of classification that is unambiguous, universally valid, and therapeutically significant (as well as scientifically reproducible). We believe that this effectively disposes of the claim that Chinese medicine is "strictly empirical," since surely such a vast body of knowledge could not have been accumulated by even the most pains-taking observation over the course of two millennia without some sort of *a priori* theoretical foundation.

The Practice of Chinese Diagnostic Medicine

THE preceding discussion of the symptoms associated with the various diagnostic criteria has already given us some idea of what the Chinese doctor is looking for when he begins to examine his patient. And, as we have seen, the simplest way of approaching this process is by means of the four traditional categories—visual inspection (*inspectio, wangzhen*), hearing and smell (*ausculatio et olfactio, wénzhen*), questioning the patient directly (*interrogatio, wènzhen*), and touching the patient's body (*palpatio, qiezhen*). By far the most important of the various *inspectiones* that the doctor might perform is the examination of the patient's tongue, though any striking superficial alteration on the surface of the patient's body will be duly noted, particular attention being paid to the eyes and ears, the teeth and gums, and the head and neck in general. (Visual examination of the patient's bodily motions and gestures, general demeanor, and bodily secretions would also be included in this first category.) The objects of the doctor's oral and olfactory examination would include the patient's voice and speech as well as the sound of his breathing, plus belching, coughing, hiccuping, and other audible symptoms of distress, where present, the smell of his breath, sweat (and other bodily secretions), and even the smell of the air in the sickroom. The patient can provide information about specific pains and functional disorders (insomnia, loss of appetite, hearing impairment, irregular menstrual periods) that might not otherwise be apparent. Finally, *palpatio* is largely a matter of examining the relevant impulse points and taking the patient's pulse, which is the most important as well as generally the last of these procedures to be carried out.

The maxim we quoted earlier that *The Yellow Prince's Classic* attributed to the celebrated physician Bian Que certainly suggests that this was not always the case (see pages 82–83) and that at one time an extremely thorough visual examination was the *sine qua non* of the

182   diagnostic art. The practice of taking the patient's pulse had apparently already been introduced, but the pulse diagnostic did not really evolve into anything like its present form until about six centuries later (c. A.D. 400). If we add to that another thirteen hundred years of gradual evolution, of increasing subtlety and refinement, then we have a total of over a hundred generations of clinical experience and a definitive diagnostic standard by which other findings can be evaluated and either confirmed or found wanting. (As compared with visual inspection or with *interrogatio,* for example, the pulse diagnostic is more precise than the former and more reliable than the latter, in the sense that it provides accurate, objective information that is presumably not subject to distortion or deliberate falsification by the patient.)

All this being the case, we will be concentrating almost exclusively on pulse diagnosis in the following discussion of diagnostic technique. (Readers who are curious about other diagnostic procedures employed in Chinese medicine are referred to the Notes at the end of this book.)[7] The pulse diagnosis might be thought of as the qualitative equivalent of laboratory tests, X rays, EKGs, or similarly definitive diagnostic tests in the repertory of Western medicine. A Western doctor will also base his diagnosis initially on a visual and tactile examination of the patient and on the patient's responses to his questions, but the doctor will naturally prefer to have these findings confirmed by one or more of these more precise standardized procedures.

THE OBJECTIVITY AND REPLICABILITY OF THE PULSE DIAGNOSTIC

These were first called into question in Japan, where Chinese medicine was adopted with very few modifications until the seventeenth century. At that time there arose a school of thought that flatly denied that (to paraphrase somewhat) the pulse diagnosis was either objective or reproducible (and thus scientifically verifiable); the technique they proposed in its stead involved palpation of the patient's chest and abdomen and is accordingly referred to as *Bauchdiagnose* or "belly diagnosis" in Western works on the subject.[8] In more recent years in China—during the Cultural Revolution, in fact—a less sweeping modification of the classical pulse diagnostic (which had never been entirely rooted out of the standard medical school curriculum) was proposed; the discipline would be "simplified" by reducing the twenty-eight or thirty iconograms (pulse patterns) recognized by classical Chinese medicine to a mere eight or ten. "Modern" doctors (i.e., those who had been trained primarily in Western medicine) objected that the pulse diagnostic should simply be permitted to wither away of its own accord, rather than artificially revived and rejuvenated. In most cases the basis of this objection was nothing more profound than ignorance and prejudice, though there were also those who advanced the fox-and-the-grapes-style argument that it was just as well that the pulse diagnostic was nothing but a pseudoscientific sham, since it was all much too difficult to learn in any case. The answer to this objection, insofar as it deserves one, is that, practically speaking, pulse diagnosis requires nothing more than the sort of presence of mind and attention to detail that we customarily expect of any competent doctor. The reluctance of a great many others (besides Chinese medical students) to recognize pulse diagnosis as a valid medical procedure is a problem of an entirely different order, however, involving as it does a number of technical and psychological issues that we would like to discuss for a moment. The central difficulty concerns the problem of objectivity; both the critics and even some of the partisans of Chinese medicine insist that the pulse diagnosis is a strictly subjective procedure (even more emphatically than is the case with other aspects of Chinese medicine). We believe this proposition to be entirely false—insofar as it can be said to have any meaning at all.

In fact, we believe it to be based on a totally mistaken notion of objectivity (though one that has found particular favor in the world of Western medicine). Ostensibly all diagnostic findings—all the essential ones, at any rate—are said to be objective (or, to be more precise, "objectifiable"—which means that they are capable of being independently ["intersubjectively"] verified in every detail). But the fact is that in medicine (including Western medicine) the vast majority of assertions that concern diagnostic findings or human disorders are neither objective nor objectifiable in the strictest sense. Clearly, psychic disorders—neuroses, phobias, etc.—in themselves are not objective (in the sense that anyone other than the subject could experience them in exactly the same way or even provide an "intersubjective" confirmation of their presence), nor are the numerous painful sensations that accompany a great many illnesses, though these can readily be distinguished from one another and qualitatively differentiated with little difficulty. This entire subjective aspect of illness is neither objective nor objectifiable by definition, though it is nevertheless of critical importance. A patient who is doubled over with pain and gasping for breath is going to want his doctor to "do something" for him in a hurry, irrespective of the fact that his symptoms are (thus far) neither objective nor objectifiable.

184   And even the sort of data that actually are objectifiable (a patient's temperature reading, for example) are generally acquired by nonobjective means in clinical practice. We have been using the word *objective* to mean "free from subjective bias, capable of being independently verified by a second observer." But when a nurse in a hospital ward takes twenty patients' temperatures between the hours of six and seven every morning and marks their charts accordingly, her findings *may* be objectifiable, but they can be truly objective only if one or more competent persons accompany her on her rounds and confirm these readings in each case. And by the same token, presumably, if three or ten or even fifty competent observers reach exactly the same conclusion after feeling the same patient's pulse, their findings may also (indeed, they must) be recognized as both objective and objectifiable.

Where quantitative data are concerned, the first prerequisites for objectivity are, of course, the accuracy of the instruments being used and the competency of whomever is taking the readings. In the case of a qualitative procedure like pulse diagnosis, the main prerequisite is the technical ability and manual dexterity. of the diagnostician. Over the course of nearly a decade as a teacher and practitioner of pulse diagnosis (both in Europe and in East Asia) I have observed that there are a number of extremely serious pedagogical pitfalls the student may encounter as he approaches technical competency. The process is somewhat similar to that of learning Braille—in both cases the student must cultivate the sensitivity of his fingertips, must learn to make very subtle tactile distinctions and also to interpret these strictly tactile stimuli as meaningful bits of information. In addition, however, let us suppose that the student is also learning to read Braille texts in an unknown language he has never heard a word of in his life and also that these texts are almost entirely concerned with a subject he has hitherto remained ignorant of. It might well happen in such a case that though the basic skills required could be picked up in months, a thorough mastery of the subject could be acquired only over several decades, and until that time a great deal of the information that he came into contact with would remain quite unintelligible to him.

The discipline of *pulsiconography,* as we shall call it, represents over two thousand years of clinical experience distilled, clarified, and refined for the benefit of today's student. This is a process that could scarcely be duplicated *ab ovo* in the course of a single lifetime, let alone hastily reconstructed by means of a few weeks' or months' instruction. Just as the student of Braille will have already thoroughly assimilated the grammar and vocabulary of his own language and even as the beginning violinist should be able to distinguish a melody from a random assemblage of sounds, in the same way the student of pulse diagnosis should have already mastered the rational discipline of pulsiconography as well as the underlying medical theory before attempting to acquire the technical skills involved. Only then will he really know what to look for when he examines a patient's pulse, and only then will he realize what he has found when he finds it. (This may seem like an elementary point, but a great many courses in pulse diagnosis have come to nothing in the end because the participants, though inspired by the best intentions and otherwise excellently qualified, hoped somehow to evade this basic prerequisite.)

There can be no doubt that a real mastery of pulse diagnosis requires an extended period of practical, hands-on instruction—just as one can hardly learn to read Braille by memorizing a printed card with a list of characters overnight. However, there are really no esoteric or special skills involved; about all that is necessary is a set of fingertips that have not been desensitized by too much manual labor (even a few hours of tennis, rowing, or puttering around in the garden are enough to desensitize one's fingers for quite some time). And finally, to make explicit what we have been assuming all along, the pulse diagnosis is no less "objective" or intersubjectively verifiable than a blind man's ability to read a Braille text correctly merely by passing his fingers over it.

Before we begin our discussion, however, we feel obliged to address ourselves to the durable legend that the pulse diagnosis had its real origins in the prudery of Chinese doctors (or the misplaced modesty of their female patients). It is true that the Chinese traditionally regarded one's clothing as an essential expression of one's personality (and are thus reluctant to cast it aside unnecessarily), and it is also true that the naked human form was almost never represented in classical Chinese art. But at no time in history did this attitude prevent conscientious Chinese doctors from examining their patient's bodies, women as well as men. A single glance at any of the classical works on acupuncture makes it clear that a great many important impulse points were to be found in areas that would normally be covered by the patient's clothing. "Male midwives" (*accoucheurs* is the more technical term) also assisted women in childbirth. In short, there is absolutely no reason to suppose that the adoption of the pulse diagnosis or the preeminent place it has come to assume in Chinese medicine was in any way motivated by some kind of seraglio mentality or an excess of moral *pudeur*.

186 *PULSES AND PULSE PATTERNS*

First, a brief review of basic terminology may be in order. We have already mentioned that the three most important pulse points (singular and plural, *situs*) are to be found on the wrist—to be precise, along the radial artery just in front of, directly over, and behind the *processus styloides radii.* (This location is also called the *ostium pollicare, cunkou* in Chinese, both of which mean "opening of the thumb.") The three radial pulse points on each hand are referred to as *pulsus pollicaris, pulsus clausalis,* and *pulsus pedalis,* after their Chinese names *cun* ("thumb"), *guan* ("a narrow pass"), and *chi* ("foot"); the first is so called because of its proximity to the thumb, the second as a fanciful description of the site itself, the third because this pulse point corresponds to the "lower regions" of the body. The basic diagnostic significance of the pulse points is that each of them is directly or indirectly correlated with one or more of the function circles (directly in the case of the storage circles, indirectly in the case of the passage circle).

Each individual pulse can be qualitatively characterized in terms of its apparent length, breadth, and depth. "Depth" in this case is described in terms of three different levels—superficial, intermediate, and "on the bone," which refers to a pulse that can be detected only by means of a relatively strong finger pressure. In addition, the principal pulse patterns may be further defined as strong or weak, "rough" (uneven), "twisted," and fast or slow (with respect to the patient's respiration rate). We would like to examine the individual pulse patterns one by one and to describe both their qualitative characteristics and their possible pathological significance, which should also give a fairly clear idea of the considerable degree of diagnostic differentiation involved in pulse diagnosis.

1. *Pulsus superficialis* (superficial pulse) can be detected on the superficial level with only a slight finger pressure. This pulse gets weaker as the pressure is increased and returns to its original strength as soon as the pressure is released. A superficial pulse is regarded as a *species* symptom; in particular, a strong superficial pulse indicates a *repletio speciei* and a weak superficial pulse an *inanitas speciei.*

2. *Pulsus mersus* (deep pulse) is to be found only "beneath the flesh," i.e., with a strong finger pressure, and is accordingly classified as an *intima* symptom. (*Species* and *intima* are used here in their original senses of "toward the surface" and "away from the surface of the body," respectively. An *intima* disorder is generally considered to be the more serious of the two.) As

before, a strong deep pulse indicates a *repletio* and a weak pulse an *inanitas*.

3. *Pulsus tardus* (slow pulse) is defined, in an adult, as fewer than four pulse beats for every breath and is associated with *algor*.

4. *Pulsus celer* (rapid pulse), more than five pulse beats for every breath, is invariably interpreted as a sign of *calor*.

5. *Pulsus inanis* (depleted pulse) is a weak pulse that can be located only after a careful examination and, once found, will disappear immediately if pressure is either increased or relaxed. In general, this indicates a departure from orthopathy in the direction of *inanitas,* and since in Chinese medicine the correct maintenance of orthopathy takes precedence over the treatment of heteropathy, it is especially important that such an elusive diagnostic indicator as this one be detected and accurately interpreted.

6. *Pulsus repletus* (overflowing pulse) is readily apparent with even the slightest finger pressure and is not abated as the pressure is increased. It is, of course, associated with *repletio*.

7. *Pulsus lubricius* (slippery pulse) is described as smooth and intermittent, feeling something like a round, slippery object beneath the skin. It is a sign of *calor repletionis* (*calor* that occurs simultaneously with a local overabundance of physiological energy) and is classified as a *yang* pulse as well, which "lets *xue* build up to its full capacity." In women it is regarded as a sign of pregnancy, assuming that no pathological symptoms are present.

8. *Pulsus asper* (rough pulse) is described as rough and intermittent, as though it were being goaded or urged on roughly—also likened to the scraping of a thin blade on a piece of bamboo. In contrast to the preceding, it is associated with depleted reserves of *xue,* individual-specific constructive energy.

9. *Pulsus longus* (long pulse) is said to be "grown out at the head and tail," which means that it is broader than a finger's breadth and thus overlaps the *situs* where it is to be found. (Chinese doctors use three fingers to examine a patient's pulse—the middle finger, index finger, and generally the ring finger as well). The long pulse is always taken as a sign of a healthy abundance of physiological energy and thus of a propitious balance of energy production and consumption.

10. *Pulsus brevis* (short pulse) is said to be "clipped at the head and tail," since it is shorter than a finger's breadth. A strong, short

pulse is a sign of an accumulation of an unreleased buildup of *qi,* individual-specific active energy and a weak, short pulse as a sign that the body's reserves of *qi* are depleted.

11. *Pulsus exudans* (surging pulse) has a rhythm that is likened to a tidal wave—at one moment exceptionally strong, then gradually ebbing away to almost nothing. This pulse pattern is taken as a sign of *calor vigens* ("thriving" or abundant *calor*).

11a. *Pulsus magnus* (great pulse) is similar to the preceding and not always distinguished from it in the medical literature. However, since the great pulse is always a symptom of an advanced heteropathy, it is not without diagnostic significance of its own.

12. *Pulsus evanescens* (disappearing pulse), as the name implies, is an extremely weak pulse and is difficult to locate. To the examining fingers it will feel like the faintest suggestion of a pulse, and from time to time it may disappear altogether. The *pulsus evanescens* is a symptom of a severe deficiency of *yang* energy and thus of a serious *inanitas.*

13. *Pulsus intentus* (taut pulse) feels tense and vibrant, like a rope that has been pulled taut. This is an *algor* symptom, and it indicates that the digestive processes have come to a complete halt; it is often accompanied by pain. In the presence of other evidence of a predominance of *yin* in the body, it also indicates the presence of a constructive heteropathy.

14. *Pulsus languidus* (relaxed pulse) is associated with *humor* and thus in turn with the function circle of the spleen and the transformation phase of earth. (A superabundance of *humor* also restricts the normal release of active energy.) This pulse generally has the normal rhythm of four beats to every breath, though it may be more sluggish at times.

15. *Pulsus chordalis* (stringy pulse) is described as being "sharp and taut like a lutestring" and is extremely long and narrow, firm and tight like its namesake. The *pulsus chordalis* is a *ventus* symptom, often accompanied by pain, and typically indicates a disorder of the function circle of the liver.

16. *Pulsus cepacaulicus* (onion-stem pulse) is a broad, long, superficial pulse that is so called because it is said to be "hollow in the middle," like the stem of a green onion. In fact, the examiner's finger will encounter a sort of gap or hiatus in the middle of this pulse where the pulsebeat intermittently disappears and

can be retrieved only by applying more pressure. The *pulsus*
cepacaulicus is a sign of the loss of *yin* energy, which might be
due to loss of blood or merely to the depletion of any of the
other forms of constructive energy.

17. *Pulsus tympanicus* (drumhead pulse) is a superficial pulse that
feels both tight and hollow to the touch, like a taut drumhead.
This indicates a serious deficiency of *xue,* which may also be
due to a considerable loss of blood, such as after childbirth, for
example, or as the result of a miscarriage.

18. *Pulsus fixus* (clinging pulse) is a long, robust, very deep pulse
that appears to be actually attached to the bone, hence its name.
This pulse is a symptom of constructive *algor,* which may lead
to a *repletio*. A patient who exhibits this pulse pattern may also
be suffering from painful abdominal cramps.

19. *Pulsus mollis* (soft pulse) is similar to the preceding but
somewhat broader and longer. It is also a symptom of *inanitas*.

20. *Pulsus invalidus* (sickly pulse) is a deep pulse but invariably thin
and thready. It is a symptom of *inanitas* of both active and
constructive energy, generally accompanied by a feeling of
weakness.

21. *Pulsus diffluens* (melting pulse) is a weak, superficial pulse that
appears to "melt away" as soon as the examiner's finger touches
it. When pressure is increased, it will disappear altogether. This
is a symptom of a decline in the body's reserves of innate
constitutional energy. If the examiner is unable to discern a
distinct outline to this pulse, then the energy of all the function
circles is already seriously depleted.

22. *Pulsus minutus* (frail pulse) is fine and thin, like a silken thread,
but it can be felt clearly and distinctly at any one of the three
levels. It is a symptom of *inanitas* of the body's reserves of both
active and constructive energy, possibly as the result of excessive
physical exertion, which may eventually deplete the energy of
the function circle of the kidneys as well. This may also be the
result of mental or emotional strain—*reflectio* or *sollicitudo*
(anxiety)—or of the influence of *humor* ("dampness") on the
circulation of energy throughout the body.

22a. *Pulsus parvus* (little pulse) is short and narrow and may be felt
on any of the three levels. It is also an *inanitas* symptom.

23. *Pulsus surreptus* (stealthy pulse) is a very deep pulse that is said
to "creep along" and can be felt only by applying the greatest

possible pressure. Even then, this pulse can be felt only intermittently, and it is a sign that physiological energy has been diverted by a heteropathy—a *repletio* symptom, in other words—and is often accompanied by severe pain.

24. *Pulsus mobilis* (moving pulse) is a strong pulse that is invariably both *lubricius* (slippery) and *celer* (rapid) as well; it is said to feel like a bean or a pod of some sort bending back and forth (very slightly, to be sure) at the end of a stalk. This is a sign that the body's active and constructive energy reserves are not harmoniously balanced.

25. *Pulsus agitatus* (racing pulse) is a very rapid pulse that appears to stop altogether at irregular intervals. It is a sign of *repletio caloris* and thus of pathological accumulations of energy in certain areas, which may be accompanied by painful swellings.

26. *Pulsus haesitans* (hanging pulse) is a sluggish pulse of intermediate strength that appears to stop altogether at irregular intervals. This is a sign of *yin vigens* ("thriving," or abundant, *yin*) and thus of a stagnant accumulation of energy, so that the normal circulation of energy is blocked to some extent (which is also accompanied by mucus congestion and constipation).

27. *Pulsus intermittens* (intermittent pulse) appears to stop completely at *regular* intervals and for a considerable period of time. This is an indication that the energy of the relevant function circle is being dangerously depleted or has already been exhausted; it may also be a symptom of *ventus*. This pulse pattern is found in patients who have sustained severe contusions or puncture wounds or possibly a very severe emotional trauma.

28. *Pulsus concitatus* (furious pulse) is an extremely agitated pulse (in adults, seven to eight pulse beats for every breath). This indicates that *yin* is almost exhausted, whereas *yang* is in a state of considerable excitation, which threatens an immediate exhaustion of *qi primum,* the body's innate reserves of energy.

SIMPLIFICATION OF THE PULSE PATTERNS

Clearly it would require considerable time and effort to acquire a complete practical mastery of this complex and difficult subject. And it is well known that the officials in the People's Republic who establish public health policy, especially in recent years, have tended to be pragmatists rather than purists, concerned with providing decent medical care for as many people in as many different localities as possible. The famous "barefoot doctors"—workers or (more frequently) farm laborers trained as paramedical auxiliaries—represent one aspect of this policy that has attracted a great deal of attention in the West. We have already mentioned the "simplified" system of pulsiconography that was introduced into the standard medical school curricula several years ago and that consists in its simplest version of only eight patterns arranged in four complementary pairs (deep and superficial, rapid and slow, full and depleted, rough and slippery). One can readily understand that the Chinese authorities are primarily concerned with what is currently called health care delivery rather than pedagogical rigor or even with traditional medicine as such. Admittedly, since the reasons for this innovation are basically political, one must also recognize that the simplified pulsiconography actually involves a renunciation of the full spectrum of diagnostic possibility that was offered by the classical system—an adulteration, if you will, of the inductive-synthetic method of Chinese medicine, which, like Western medicine, has always striven for greater precision and a higher level of differentiation rather than the reverse.

And since this policy change has naturally been reflected in the content of the standard Chinese medical texts, this also means that the Western doctor who is interested in investigating traditional Chinese medicine directly from the primary sources is actually going to be confronted in all likelihood with this drastically modified (and considerably Westernized) version of the classical system of pulsiconography. Clearly, though, a Western doctor is unlikely to be interested in a crash course in what is essentially another variety of "nuts and bolts" basic medicine (as purveyed by the latest Chinese textbooks) when instead what is required is a supplement to, rather than a substitute for, what we already have, something that can fill in the gaps that conventional Western medicine has so far been unable to.

In reality, however, equally or even more drastically simplified systems of pulsiconography are currently in use among Western acupuncturists. Gerhard Bachmann, one of the pioneers of the discipline in northern Europe, refers to only six different pulse patterns, and other writers make do with even fewer than that.[9] There would seem to be some justification for this, at least, since classical acu-moxa-therapy itself uses only three pulse patterns: the superficial, deep, and full pulses (and the latter two, regarded as *intima* symptoms, only indirectly and under certain circumstances). According to Chinese medical theory, acupuncture can do nothing to renew the body's depleted energy reserves, though

192   it may be helpful in draining off excess energy, in breaking up abnormal concentrations of energy, in unblocking congested arterial pathways, and generally in restoring a harmonious distribution of energy throughout the body. Thus, if pulse diagnosis reveals *inanitas* symptoms exclusively, then acupuncture would be categorically ruled out. And, once again, it is our belief that the therapist who really wants to explore the full spectrum of diagnostic possibility (even where acu-moxa-therapy is concerned) should be acquainted with a far greater number of pulse patterns (let us say twenty, in fact).

This brings us to the more fundamental question of whether, within the context of Chinese traditional medicine as presented in these pages so far, any attempt at simplifying the classical pulsiconography is justifiable or even desirable. Once again assuming that we are concerned here with the public health problems of the industrialized nations of the West (rather than those of the People's Republic of China or any of the other developing countries that have chosen to follow their lead in encouraging a revival of traditional medicine), then, quite simply, we believe the answer to be no. As we see it (and as we have tried to make clear in our opening chapter), the most critical deficiency of modern Western medicine is qualitative rather than quantitative, namely, the inability of otherwise highly competent physicians to treat certain chronic, congenital, psychic, and functional disorders except with merely palliative or nonspecific measures. It seems clear that the successful treatment of such congenital or chronic (including a great many "psychosomatic") disorders would require a highly differentiated, exact, and highly specific diagnostic method—and certainly not some sort of exotic or primitive "alternative medicine." The subtlety and high degree of differentiation that Chinese medicine has acquired from two thousand years of clinical experience is not just empty pedantry or diagnostic hair-splitting; this may well represent the optimal (even perhaps the minimal) level of completeness and complexity that is necessary to arrive at a clinical picture of an illness that is both rational and effective.

THE PROBLEM OF IDENTIFYING PULSE PATTERNS BY MECHANICAL MEANS

Suppose it has been decided that Chinese diagnostic methods, the pulse diagnosis in particular, should immediately be introduced into clinical practice in the West. In that case, should there also be some attempt to provide an appropriate instrument that could identify pulse patterns automatically, "objectively" (to revert to the terms of our previous discussion a few pages earlier)? We have already had quite a bit to say about the objectivity of the pulse diagnostic as it is currently practiced; this new supposition raises two additional questions: whether such a procedure would be technically feasible and whether it might have a legitimate clinical application.

Successful experiments along these lines have been carried out for several decades now and have demonstrated that it is technically possible to identify individual pulse patterns with a high degree of accuracy. The simplest of these devices is very simple indeed, the most complex no less so than those electronic scanners that are currently going into production that can "read" a printed text entirely by themselves. In short, the problem is as good as solved, but the question remains whether there would be a genuine clinical need for any of these devices. As we have already tried to make clear, one of Chinese medicine's greatest strongpoints is its *comprehensibility*—both in the sense of clarity and also in the sense of its relative simplicity and "compactness," the fact that it is not so vast in scope that it cannot be grasped in its entirety by an individual human mind. This latter quality is at least partially due to the fact that even in an extremely complicated case a diagnosis can generally be arrived at in less than two hours; most disorders can be diagnosed in less than one hour, proceeding very carefully and taking all relevant data into account. This not only means that a skillful diagnostician is less likely to overlook something important but also that, since all the facts in the case will pass before his eyes in such a short time, it will be that much simpler for him to decide which of them are really relevant. It takes the average student about four years to acquire a thorough grounding in traditional Chinese medicine, of which about three to six months, at most, are devoted to the acquisition of the degree of manual dexterity and sensitivity that is necessary to make an accurate pulse diagnosis. And—to reiterate once more—the real value of the pulse diagnosis as a source of clinical data is not so much a function of the skill of the individual practitioner as of the accumulated, and progressively refined, clinical experience of two thousand years.

What would be gained by entrusting this task to an electronic monitor? First, an entirely new pulsiconography would have to be worked out, not only by the manufacturers of the device but by the prospective users as well. (Even the "meaning" of an EEG or an EKG is not self-evident; their interpretation requires considerable training—and incidentally, in contrast to the Chinese pulsiconogram, which can provide a variety of highly detailed information about all the function

194   circles, the inferences that can be drawn from them are limited in scope.) And this means that the time the student would have to devote simply to mastering the instrument would be all that much greater, though at present there can be no guarantee that the margin of error would be any less with an electronic monitor. Thus there would most probably be a considerable reduction in accuracy and precision for the first few decades that the new system was in place, to say nothing of the expenditure of time, money, and effort that would be involved.

Though in exceptional cases an individual pulse diagnosis may require more than an hour to carry out, the average is closer to ten minutes. And the instrumentality involved—the experienced diagnostician—is available at any hour of the day or night, highly mobile, and fully capable of evaluating not only the depth, length, and breadth of a pulse at any *situs* but also of observing the presence or absence of a ringlike formation (a so-called *halo*) around the pulse point, a torsion or twisting of the artery, and a great deal else besides. This includes an evaluation of the minute anatomical peculiarities of the *situs* itself, which will never be quite the same in any two individuals. There are sex-linked variations that depend on the relative flexibility of the subcutaneous fatty tissue and on typical differences in bodily proportions between men and women; men's pulse points, for example, tend to be relatively short as compared to women's. Finally, there are subtle differences between the pulse patterns exhibited in infancy, youth, and adulthood that also have to be taken into account, as well as long-term "interference patterns" associated with certain ecological factors, medium-term effects of local climatic conditions, and the short-term, transitory effects of consuming certain foods or stimulants.

Experienced diagnosticians can also distinguish almost immediately between information that is of real value and information that is not really relevant in formulating a diagnosis—something that even the most sophisticated artificial intelligence is only just beginning to be able to do and that is of course well beyond the capacity of the sort of electronic devices we are talking about here. If this winnowing process has to be performed after the fact, by examining a sheaf of printout rather than the patient's wrists, then the time and expense will be correspondingly greater, even though this procedure itself lacks the inherent rigor, reliability, and cogency of the traditional method. To summarize, then, the great achievement of classical Chinese medicine is not so much reflected in the doctor's skill in examining the patient's pulse—in obtaining the requisite diagnostic data—as in his ability to apply a precise, highly differential, and fully reproducible method of interpreting these data. An electronic "pulsiconograph" may be capable of taking over this first task, but for the foreseeable future the second will still have to be left entirely to a human diagnostician.

VARIABILITY OF NORMAL PULSE PATTERNS

In Chinese medicine, the concept of a "normal pulse" is a purely theoretical one, an idealized construct of the sort that is never actually encountered in practice. Every individual's pulse is unique, and in most cases the pulse will exhibit certain distinct peculiarities—congenital or constitutional, age- or sex-linked, climatic or seasonal—and thus various functional predispositions or tendencies as well. These are of particular interest to the diagnostician, since they permit certain inferences to be drawn about the sort of external factors or influences that might cause these normal functional tendencies to become pathological or that, on the other hand, might enhance the body's natural resistance.

There is a definite correlation between the so-called endomorphic or pyknic (fleshy) physical type and the deep pulse pattern, likewise between the asthenic or ectomorphic (spare, slender) physical type and the superficial pulse. A very active individual is likely to exhibit a surging pulse (*pulsus exudans*) or great pulse (*pulsus magnus*) at all six pulse points, though this is to be regarded simply as a sign of normal good health, and even the most scrupulous examination may fail to detect any other "pathological" symptoms. The sort of person that a seventeenth-century physician would have described as "sanguine"—ruddy, robust, possibly short-tempered as well—may normally exhibit a relaxed pulse (*languidus*), while the "phlegmatic" physical type—heavyset, stolid—is associated with the frail pulse (*minutus*). Every experienced pulse diagnostician can testify to the fact that the pulse patterns of all the inhabitants of a particular locality are likely to have certain characteristic "overtones" in common; a striking example of this phenomenon, at least in temperate climates, is provided by the change in the seasons. In Central Europe the *pulsus chordalis* (stringy pulse), described as being long, narrow, and "taut as a lutestring," is more common in springtime, when the body's reserves of energy have been freshly replenished. In summer the pulse typically becomes longer and broader and appears to move toward the surface—the *pulsus exudans* (surging pulse) pattern—and in fall this latter tendency becomes even more pronounced (*pulsus superficialis*). In winter, on the other hand, the deep pulse (*pulsus mersus*) tends to predominate.

196   What is more, in these days of routine jet travel it is possible to make direct comparisons of the pulse patterns of inhabitants of different global climatic zones. The inhabitants of the Arctic regions tend, as one might expect, to have deeper pulses; the inhabitants of the tropics to have broader, superficial pulses. This also provides a simple test for establishing whether an intercontinental traveler has been properly acclimated to his temporary place of residence, or whether he has under- or overcompensated or even (as a pathological reaction to the change of climate and circumstances) exhibits a completely anomalous pulse pattern.

An individual with a sedentary occupation who does not otherwise get much exercise will generally exhibit a sickly pulse (*invalidus*) at the distal *situs* (the pulse point nearest the thumb, also referred to as the *pulsus pollicaris*), even though there may well be no other abnormal symptoms of any kind. Someone who leads an especially strenuous life—an athlete, for example—is likely to have a rapid, "enlarged" pulse (*pulsus celer sive pulsus magnus*). The *pulsus pedalis* (at the proximal *situs,* the most distant from the base of the thumb) may also disclose more intimate information about the individual's manner of life. A sickly pulse at this pulse point, which is associated with prolonged sexual continence, is called the "true monk's pulse" by Chinese doctors, since it was regarded as an infallible test for distinguishing between the genuine celibate and the brother who had been leading a less disciplined sort of life outside the monastery gates. A particularly vigorous sex life is said to result in a superficial pulse at this *situs,* perhaps even a frail (*minutus*) or depleted (*inanis*) pulse— though these latter two are almost to be regarded as symptoms of an aberration of some kind.

Diet and the use of stimulants will also affect the individual's pulse pattern, which is why a Chinese doctor will prefer to take a patient's pulse immediately after he wakes up in the morning, and before he has had anything to eat. In extremely serious or problematical cases this procedure is always observed, though as a rule an experienced diagnostician can successfully isolate any "overtones" in the pulse pattern associated with the consumption of certain foods. In addition, the pulse at the medial *situs* tends to be sickly (*invalidus*) after a short fast, superficial or depleted after a longer fast; if the patient eats something at this point, this will eventually result in a surging (*exudans*) or relaxed (*languidus*) pulse at the medial *situs*. Drinking coffee or alcohol has an almost instantaneous effect on the distal pulse, which tends to speed up and to become "enlarged." Habitual consumption of these substances may also result in abnormal perturbations of the *clusalis* pulse.

In an age when practically every patient who visits a doctor's office (to say nothing of a hospital) ends up taking some sort of medication, it is of overriding importance for a doctor who administers any drug to be able to determine, clearly and unequivocally, whether or not the patient is responding properly to treatment (and whether or not the patient is able to tolerate the side effects of the drug). The practitioner of Chinese medicine also has to decide whether the chemical medication that a colleague has prescribed for one of his patients is working at cross-purposes with the course of treatment that he himself has decided on. Pulsiconography can answer both of these questions directly. If the underlying disorder has caused a "narrowing" of the patient's pulse and the medication has caused it to become narrower still, then the treatment has unquestionably caused the patient's condition to deteriorate—he may even be in some danger at this point. If the patient's pulse has gotten "broader" and more relaxed as a result of the treatment, then this is definitely a sign that the treatment has been effective (though only one of many such signs, to be sure).

A quite different problem is presented by the sort of medication that has no medicinal effects of its own (i.e., it does not cause the physiological function in question to shift perceptibly in one direction or the other) but whose sole purpose is to help counteract the sort of havoc that might be wreaked by more potent medication. The immediate effect of this auxiliary medication may be the appearance of the moving pulse (*pulsus mobilis*), characterized as shorter and more rapid, "slippery" and superficial. In Chinese medical theory this phenomenon is explained as the result of dissonance or dissension between active impulses and constructive restraint, which seems to fit the case very neatly. The *pulsus mobilis* may also be the result of an overdose or the administration of an inappropriate medication—or a reaction to a particular food that the patient is unable to tolerate. When accompanied by all the usual symptoms of a highly acute digestive disorder, its presence should alert the doctor that the patient who is "not currently on any medication" is telling less than the entire truth.

SUMMARY: THE ROLE OF PULSICONOGRAPHY AS A DIAGNOSTIC TOOL

Even though the foregoing sketch can hardly do justice to the complexity of the subject, we hope that we have at least established a few of the more basic points: The classical pulse diagnostic can be regarded as a collection of well-organized and readily verifiable principles that can enable the

198   practitioner to distinguish what is medically significant from what is merely routine or ephemeral amid the vast profusion of physiological impulses and alterations that mark the passage of our lives as individuals. As a diagnostic technique, it is unrivaled among all the varieties of medicine currently being practiced for its completeness, rigor, and effectiveness. To reject it out of hand simply because it requires a modest amount of manual training on the part of the practitioner (and no more than the normal quotient of attentiveness to detail and mental acuity) is comparable, let us say, to refusing to learn to play a musical instrument because any given tone you might eventually be able to produce can already be synthesized electronically (and almost anything you might care to play is already available on records or tapes). It should not be necessary to point out that the current crisis in Western medicine has a great deal to do with this attitude of totally irrational skepticism—of just the sort that might induce one to reject a method that is simple and perfectly reliable in favor of another that is more respectable and ruinously expensive, as well as untried, unverifiable, and severely limited in its application.

VI

THERAPY

Therapeutic Techniques

A SUITABLE introduction to the subject, in the form of a dialogue between the Yellow Prince and the Count of Qi, is provided in *The Yellow Prince's Classic:*

THE PRINCE: I should like to hear about the essential path of healing.

THE COUNT: Most important of all, you must never go astray in your evaluation of the patient's color [physical appearance] and pulse, and then you must make good use of what you have observed. That is the one great rule of healing. When the elements of *contravectio* ["running against the current"] and *secundovectio* ["running with the current"] are promiscuously mixed together, when one does not fully grasp either the superficial or the essential aspects, then the constellational force is dissipated, and one loses his mastery. To forsake what is played out and take up what is new, that is the way to become accomplished.

THE PRINCE: Now I have heard from you what is truly essential. But what you have said to me only has to do with color and pulse, and I already know perfectly well how important they are.

THE COUNT: The perfection of healing is the One.

THE PRINCE: And what is that?

THE COUNT: It may be found by seeking out the agents of disease.

THE PRINCE: And how would I go about doing that?

THE COUNT: You would close all doors and windows [i.e., shut out all distractions] and question the patient closely and logically. By this means are revealed both the patient's sensations and the special circumstances of his case—as well as its true significance [i.e., the nature of the pathological agents involved], which has thus far been concealed behind them. Whoever can truly come to grips with the constellational force in this manner will achieve success; whoever cannot will strive in vain.

THE PRINCE: Just so![1]

Like any mature medical science, Chinese medicine uses a great many highly specific remedies and treatments as well as others that are less specific. The first category includes primarily what is called *internal therapy* (*neizhi*), a diversified and highly differentiated repertory of drugs and herbal remedies, as well as *external therapy* (*naichi*), namely acupuncture and moxibustion. The less specific treatments that make up the second category play a subordinate or auxiliary role in practice, either in conjunction with a generalized program of preventive medicine or to provide a mild form of assistance to some more specific treatment. These might include massage, baths of various kinds (steam baths, inhalation of steam or medicinal vapor), *qi* exercises, and a supervised diet, as well as certain other suggested modifications in the patient's habitual mode of life.

Since earliest times the administration of remedies from this vast pharmacopoeia has been far and away the most important, the most highly diversified, and the most predictable and readily controllable of all forms of therapy employed by traditional Chinese medicine. Indeed, traditional Chinese pharmacology can easily bear comparison with modern Western drug therapy, and with regard to the richness and the subtlety of the means at its disposal as well as its rational coherence and effectiveness, Chinese pharmacology is at least the equal and in many respects the superior of its Western counterpart. Once again, the integrity of Chinese pharmacology as a systematic discipline rests on over two thousand years of clinical experience and experimentation on the basis of which the precise effects of each of these remedies has been qualitatively and unambiguously defined. The qualitative precision of this system might be likened to the tumblers of a lock, the key to which is provided by the classical Chinese diagnostic, fashioned according to the same criteria and the same normative conventions—and of course primarily concerned as well with physiological functions. We would like to examine the mechanism of the lock a little more closely now, simply to demonstrate that the therapeutic system embodied in classical Chinese medicine is not only comprehensible but also eminently practical and highly relevant to the basic conditions of our lives as human beings.

THE PRINCIPLES OF QUALITATIVE CLASSIFICATION: TEMPERATURE (XING)

In Chinese pharmacology, remedies and their effects are classified according to certain normative conventions in much the same way that symptoms are classified by means of certain diagnostic criteria. Prominent among the latter, as you may recall, are the concepts of *algor* ("cold") and *calor* ("heat"); remedies are correspondingly classified as hot, warm, cool, and cold (in addition to those that are regarded as neutral with respect to temperature). "Warm" and "hot" remedies may be used to compensate for *algor* heteropathies and to stimulate the active forms of energy; "cool" and "cold" remedies help to reduce *calor* symptoms and to dissipate *ardor* ("glowing heat," one of the six climatic excesses). Even those remedies that have no well-defined affinity with any particular temperature category are said to "raise up"—i.e., to promote—the flow of active energy toward the surface (and thus to help prevent a *species* heteropathy from penetrating deeper into the body).

REMEDIES CORRELATED WITH TASTE SENSATIONS (SAPORES)

We have already seen in our discussion of orbisiconography how each of the function circles is linked with a corresponding transformation phase as well as a characteristic taste sensation (*sapor*), the latter of which are classified, for drugs and herbal remedies as well as for food and drink, into five categories: sour, bitter, sharp, salty, and sweet. (Odorless and tasteless remedies are said to be neutral, of course.) It is important to distinguish between the *sapores* associated with the function circles, which is purely a system of conventions for describing the directional motion and the dynamic qualities of the individual circles, and the actual "flavors" that may be ascribed to particular foods or drugs. A great many Chinese remedies are also associated with more than one *sapor,* and the subtler characteristics of these remedies are said to be determined by the proportional relationships between or among the relevant *sapores.* There is clearly a difference between a remedy that is cold and sharp (like mint) and one that is hot and sharp (like most varieties of pepper), between one in which the sharpness is mitigated by other *sapores* or in which it is mingled with bitterness, for example. (This is why it is necessary for the practitioner of Chinese medicine to be aware of the *sapores* associated with a particular remedy in addition to its other dynamic properties.)

When a remedy is assigned a distinctive *sapor,* this also provides a

204   description of its effects in terms of directional motion, which is based directly on the correlation between the transformation phases and the *sapores:* sour and wood, bitter and fire, sweet and earth, sharp and metal, salty and water. (The neutral *sapor* is also associated with the transformation phase of earth.) Each of the *sapores* also has a characteristic generalized effect on the function circles; sour contracts and coalesces, stanches the flow of blood, roughens, congests; bitter dries out, depresses, subdues, or damps; sweet regulates, evens out, harmonizes, softens, buffers, and supports; sharp opens up, dissolves, and mobilizes active energy (*qi*); salty softens, moistens, and purges or purifies.

We have already learned, for example, that the transformation phase of wood is identified with activity in its highest potential stage—a quality that not only all sour *sapores* but also the function circles of the liver and gall bladder, the hours around sunset, and the springtime are all said to partake of. When we reflect on the fact that sour *sapores* have a contracting (i.e., an astringent), roughening, or constipating effect—which one need not have studied Chinese pharmacology to have observed—then it becomes clearer what is meant by a phrase like "activity in its highest potential stage." If too much energy (either active or constructive) is dissipated by a high skin temperature, excessive perspiration, diarrhea, or extreme excitability or agitation (not merely excitement), then the "tension in the bowstring" slackens or threatens to snap, the body's reserves of active energy can be released only in restricted amounts. The application of sour *sapores* may counteract this, but of course this does not imply that the remedy can be self-administered in whatever dosage or concentration seems appropriate or over however long a period as one chooses. (The result might well be a massive *repletio* brought about by this influx of fully potentiated energy, which would naturally tend to seek release in an explosive and highly disruptive manner.) A patient's idiosyncratic craving for sour *sapores* may be interpreted as an indication either that the function circles storing potential energy that is released during certain activities are not operating at full capacity or that there has actually been a considerable overproduction, resulting in a serious *repletio* of the affected circles.

THE SPECIES AND INTIMA OF PHARMACODYNAMICS: THE FOUR CHARACTERISTIC EFFECTS OF TRADITIONAL REMEDIES

In a carefully coordinated therapeutic system, precise information about the optimal dosages and therapeutic application of remedies is of course essential. The characteristic effects of a particular remedy may be evaluated in terms of a systematic and comprehensive description of the *sapores* and temperature affinities (hot, warm, cool, cold) associated with it. Chinese medicine distinguishes four conventional "tendencies," or characteristic effects, of traditional remedies:

1. "Superficial tendency" (*fu, superficialitas*). Remedies of this type (*medicamenta superficialia*) are called for when the diagnosis indicates that only the *species* region of the body is affected. This is the case, e.g., with illnesses that are acute or recent in origin. Superficial remedies are strong in *qi* and have well-defined temperature affinities, which makes them useful in controlling abnormal temperatures in the *species* region. This property is found most often in remedies that are both sweet and hot, sweet and warm, or sharp and hot; familiar examples of *medicamenta superficialia* include ginger, cinnamon, and monkshood (also known as aconite or wolfsbane).

2. "Uplifting tendency" (*elevatio*). A patient suffering from an energy deficiency in the *species* region is likely to have a low natural resistance to disease, since the body's defensive energy has been depleted, and a *species* heteropathy may easily penetrate to the interior of the body. To circumvent this, a Chinese doctor will prescribe *medicamenta elevantia,* which encourage energy that is "trapped" in the *intima* region to flow toward the surface. (Note that no additional energy is contributed by this process; available energy is merely redistributed.) "Uplifting" remedies are not particularly strong in *qi,* nor do they have sharply defined temperature affinities, which would primarily include sweet and neutral remedies as well as mildly sharp and neutral remedies, sharp and mildly warm remedies, and mildly bitter and neutral remedies.

3. "Downward-flowing tendency." *Medicamenta demittentia* are called for in the opposite case, when a surplus of *qi* has accumulated in the *species* region. In such a case, the patient's face will be unusually red and he will feel hot all over and will be sweating

lightly. This does not mean that there is an excess of *qi* throughout the body but generally that there is a local deficit of constructive energy (in the form of blood, fluids, or some other bodily substance) that normally mitigates and restricts these somewhat alarming manifestations of the active principle. Such symptoms as these are referred to as "rootless *yang* striking outward," and it would clearly be unwise to allow this energy to be dissipated. Instead its flow must be contained and redirected toward the interior of the body so that the disrupted balance of energy between *species* and *intima* may be restored. The administration of *medicamenta demittentia* can correct this imbalance and contributes indirectly to the restoration of normal *yin* functions; bleeding, which may also be taken as a sign of "rootless" or unbonded energy in the *intima* region, can also be controlled in this way. These remedies are mild-tasting for the most part and are variously classified as sweet and cold, sweet and cool, sweet and neutral, sour and neutral, and salty and neutral. The majority of these substances are actually powdered metals or minerals (e.g., magnetite, and chalk from oyster shells), though organic remedies such as *Poria* (a genus of forest mushrooms) and peony root are not infrequently encountered in practice.

4. "Deep-working tendency." There are some disturbances in the balance of the body's normal energy flow that might be likened to an explosion in a boiler or, less dramatically, to an engine overheating; these are frequently systemic in origin and entirely confined to the *intima*, the organic foundation of the function circles. These disorders are almost always accompanied by a high fever and may include such highly infectious diseases as typhus and dysentery. *Medicamenta mersa* are invariably classified as cold with a bitter or a salty *sapor;* one of the most frequently prescribed of these remedies is derived from the rhizome of *Coptis teeta,* a herb related to goldthread; others include philodendron bark, rhubarb, gentian root, and Glauber's salts (sodium sulfate), all but the first of which once occupied a prominent place in the Western pharmacopoeia as well.

THE CORRELATION BETWEEN REMEDIES AND THE INDIVIDUAL FUNCTION CIRCLES

According to Chinese medical theory, every remedy has an effect on at least one function circle (some operate specifically on only one; others have a wider spectrum of effects on various circles). Providing a complete description of the relationship between specific remedies and the function circles is the principal task of Chinese pharmacology. The doctor's examination of the patient presents the doctor with a clinical picture that corresponds to a specific heteropathy; naturally, he hopes to have a remedy at his disposal that is specifically effective against it. In Chinese the suffix *guijing* (literally, "emptying into such-and-such an arterial pathway") is used to designate a given remedy's specific correlation with a particular function circle (for which we have coined an equivalent term, *sinarteriotropic*).

The high degree of selectivity that characterizes traditional Chinese remedies—together with a remarkably detailed and reliable body of information describing their recommended dosage levels and compatibility with one another—enables the practitioner to avoid the sort of side effects that are routinely associated with Western pharmaceuticals. It is no accident that there is no equivalent expression in Chinese medicine; "side effects" can be described only in terms of "therapeutic error," an "incorrect dosage," or simply "malpractice." But, of course, not even the most skillful practitioner of Chinese pharmacology is infallible, and with a complex diagnosis that entails a complex, multistage therapeutic sequence, the initial dosage may not always be quite accurate in the case of every single ingredient in the prescription. But even then, thanks to the strictly defined relationship between diagnostic observation and the known characteristics of the various remedies, the efficacy of the prescription can be precisely tested almost immediately and the initial oversight quite easily corrected.

This ability to adapt itself to the requirements of the individual patient is one of the strongpoints of Chinese medicine. If a doctor discovers, for example, that his patient reacts abnormally to temperature—that he shivers more readily or perspires less copiously than the average person—then his treatment of this functional disorder will necessarily take into account momentary fluctuations in the outside temperature and other underlying seasonal and climatic influences. In the late morning or the late afternoon he will be more cautious in administering medication that "opens up" the *species* region (that "drives out the sweat" or, as we might say, "opens up the pores") than at other times of the day, more circumspect in prescribing these remedies at the height of summer than in the fall or winter.

Alternative Treatment Strategies: The Eight Therapeutic Methods (Bafa)

IN practice, after a doctor has completed his diagnosis and before he writes his prescription, he decides on a preliminary "treatment strategy," to be carried out by administering drugs or herbal remedies, or perhaps by other means as well. Conventionally there are eight of these: to induce sweating (*han, sudatio*), to induce vomiting (*tu, vomitio et expectoratio*), to administer a purge or a laxative (*xia, purgatio*), to harmonize antagonistic functions (*he, compositio*), to warm up the patient gradually (*wen, tepefactio*), to refresh or cool off the patient (*qing, refrigeratio*), to augment or suffuse with energy (*bu, suppletio*), and to diffuse or discharge an accumulation of energy (*xiao, xie, san; dispulsio, diffusio*). (Here we would like to issue our usual disclaimer: bear in mind that though our renderings of these terms do have some correspondence with empirical reality, they are primarily technical terms in Chinese medical theory, whose precise meanings should become somewhat clearer in the course of the following discussion. And though our equivalents for these terms may be serviceable in a broad, categorical sense, they are also likely to give rise to certain preconceptions and associations that may prove to be misleading or erroneous and that the reader is invited to disregard.)

1. *To induce sweating* (*han, sudatio*). The virtues of copious sweating have been recognized in the West in folk medicine, by the Scholastic disciples of Galen, and more recently by the adherents of naturopathy, who would contend that sweating is the way in which the body ordinarily disposes of certain waste products and other unwholesome detritus. From the Chinese perspective, though not precisely false, such a statement would seem like a crude and unscientific oversimplification. There are many different kinds of sweating, and many different reasons why it occurs. Roughly speaking, there is a different kind of sweating

that corresponds to each one of the eight leading criteria, and these must be distinguished from one another in the course of formulating a diagnosis both by questioning the patient and by direct observation.

The Chinese also recognize, of course, that sweating may also help to flush out wastes and poisons from the body—as when, for example, the patient's sweat smells especially pungent or leaves stains on his clothing, or when beads of sweat are apparent only in certain areas of the body. These phenomena are regarded as symptoms of *calor* or of a *repletio* (with respect to certain functions) or *inanitas* (with respect to others). The theory is that sweat breaks out when the equilibrium between active and constructive energy is disturbed by any of these external or internal factors, though this in itself, of course, need not be regarded as abnormal or pathological, as when one breaks out in a sweat during strenuous physical activity. Only in extreme cases of this kind (exhaustion brought on by overwork, heatstroke, or dehydration) would medical intervention be appropriate—as it would with patients suffering from chronic illnesses who have perspiration collecting in the folds of the skin or whose foreheads break out in a sweat for no apparent reason, or with terminal patients who are literally giving up the last of their vital fluids. No two of these cases would be really comparable, and only a full diagnosis could reveal whether an outbreak of sweating should be regarded as conducive or detrimental to orthopathy, whether it should be encouraged or controlled by medication or other forms of treatment.

In general, the practice of causing the patient to perspire freely (*sudatio*) is recommended only when a *repletio* in the *species* region has brought about an obstruction of the pores that interferes with normal perspiration—and only when the underlying disorder is clearly confined to the *species* region. In short, this treatment should be carried out only during the early stages of an acute illness—more specifically, when there is a finding of *algor speciei* accompanied by shivering, a slight fever, a stale taste in the mouth, a white and very moist coating on the tongue, fugitive pains in various parts of the body, and a pounding, superficial pulse, or, alternatively, if there has been a finding of *calor speciei* characterized by a high fever, slight shivering (if

any), thirst, bright red tongue with a yellowish coating, and a
rapid, superficial pulse.

2. *To induce vomiting (tu, vomitio et expectoratio)*. The Chinese
word *tu* simply means "to spit out, to spew out" (i.e., to cough
up mucus as well as to vomit up the contents of the stomach).
Such a drastic procedure may be in order when the patient is
suffering from a highly acute, life-threatening illness associated
with a severe *repletio*. Symptoms of such an illness might include
shortness of breath, a choking or suffocating feeling, incipient or
acute heart failure, apoplexy (which in Chinese medical parlance
would include the sudden failure of any major organ, including
the lungs), and extreme weakness accompanied by stertorous
breathing. In a less critical case—in which, for example, the
digestive processes have come to a complete standstill and the
patient complains of abdominal pains and a "stuffed" or
"leaden" feeling in the abdomen—the administration of an
emetic may bring about a very rapid improvement in his
condition.

In theoretical terms, this very direct and straightforward
therapeutic procedure helps to disperse abnormal, isolated
accumulations of energy and to remove certain obstructions that
may hinder or prevent the normal transmission of energy.
However, this does not mean that the doctor simply administers
an emetic or an expectorant and hopes for the best, since a
precise diagnosis and the known affinities of certain remedies for
particular function circles makes it possible to target the affected
circle or circles quite specifically.

3. *To administer a purge or a laxative (xia, purgatio)*. The use of a
purge (laxative or diuretic) is also recommended in cases of
certain highly acute disorders and is the only one of these
Chinese therapeutic techniques to have found much favor in the
West (at least among the Galenist physicians of yesteryear and
the modern naturopaths). Apart from its obvious utility in
dealing with a stubborn case of constipation (or retention of
urine), *purgatio* may also be recommended when a patient
complains of a "bloated" feeling (or appears to be suffering from
abnormal retention of water) in the abdominal region.

4. *To harmonize antagonistic functions (he, compositio)*. In contrast to
such starkly utilitarian procedures as *vomitio* and *purgatio*, this

fourth therapeutic strategy is comprehensible only in the context of Chinese medical theory. In general, it is recommended when the normal interplay among the function circles has been disrupted, though this physiological dissonance may be announced by what would seem to the layman (or the patient) to be a motley collection of symptoms: hot and cold flashes, dizzy spells, absentmindedness, dry throat, and a feeling of congestion or tightness in the chest and rib cage, as well as vomiting, loss of appetite, lassitude, and a general loss of initiative. The symptoms that would be apparent only to the examining physician exhibit a greater degree of consistency: an exceptionally unstable, streaky coating on the tongue; a narrow, elongated, superficial *chordalis* (stringy) pulse; and erratic outbreaks of perspiration, among others. All of these various symptoms of instability and irregularity may be controlled by a special class of remedies, so-called *medicamenta regulatoria*.

However, the doctor may sometimes do more harm than good by attempting to harmonize antagonistic functions. *Species* and *intima* are in opposition by their very nature, which means that in a healthy individual their functions may be thought of as interlocking harmoniously but never overlapping or intermingling. Thus, for example, if the diagnosis reveals that a disorder is confined to either of these two regions, then an ill-advised attempt to tamper with the equilibrium between the inner and outer circles is only likely to facilitate the spread of the disorder to circles that have thus far been unaffected.

5. *To warm up the patient gradually* (*wen, tepefactio*). This strategy uses remedies that serve to raise the energy level in certain function circles and is recommended for the control of *algor* symptoms. Remember from our earlier discussion of the eight leading criteria that a doctor's finding of *algor* does not necessarily imply that the patient has a chill or is physically cold. *Algor* symptoms may also include a certain sluggishness of the vital functions, a tendency toward diarrhea, and the appearance of painful permanent callosities under the skin—irrespective of the patient's subjective impressions or his actual body temperature at any given moment. This process of warming up the patient carefully and gradually is accomplished by administering remedies that are categorized as warm or hot and thus restoring the body's functional equilibrium from within.

6. *To refresh or cool off the patient* (*qing, refrigeratio*). In colloquial
Chinese the word *qing* means "clear" or "to clear up," but in
Chinese medical parlance it refers specifically to the process of
"cooling off" a *calor*-induced disorder in the *intima* region.
These come in many different varieties, and they may manifest
themselves either as primary disorders or as a consequence of
some other illness. *Calor*-induced disorders affect (or threaten)
the body's reserves of constructive energy; they act directly on
the body's physical substance—in other words, deplete the
bodily fluids—and may bring the body's essential functions
(digestion, excretion) to a standstill. Other symptoms might
include skin rashes and ulcerations, heart palpitations, extreme
agitation and irritability, loss of sensory acuity, disorientation,
and exhaustion. The pulse will always be accelerated, generally
superficial, "wide" and "surging"; the tongue may be dry, with
a yellow, gray, or black coating. Chronic *calor* disorders may
deplete the patient's bodily fluids to such an extent that he
appears gaunt and emaciated.

7. *To augment or suffuse with energy* (*bu, suppletio*). *Suppletio*
("completion") is another procedure that is unique to Chinese
medicine. The word *bu* ordinarily means "to patch up," "to fill
in," or "to mend" a hole in anything from a jacket to a
cofferdam, or more generally just "to fix" or "put right." In
Chinese medical terminology the defect that is to be remedied
is invariably an *inanitas,* usually a deficit of physiological energy
in a single function circle or functional region, occasionally a
more extensive departure from orthopathy. As you may recall,
inanitas symptoms are primarily those of fatigue or exhaustion:
lack of endurance or initiative, taciturnity, shortness of breath,
a pronounced need for sleep or rest, and a languid, apathetic
approach to life in general—though other symptoms may also
include a tendency toward excitability, anxiety and restlessness,
pallor, and ringing in the ears (tinnitus). Basically we can
imagine this process of *suppletio* as simply that of furnishing
a catalyst that mobilizes the body's hidden or latent reserves
of energy (both active and constructive) and frees them for action, the principal result of which is that the individual's
normal ability to react to external stimuli is restored as is
(indirectly) the body's ability to renew and replenish its physical
substance.

8. *To diffuse or discharge an accumulation of energy* (*xiao, xie, san; dispulsio, diffusio*). Congestion, obstruction, blockages, and stagnant accumulations of energy, wherever and in whatever form they might occur, are by far the most frequent indications or concomitants of illness. Even in cases where an *inanitas* is the primary pathological event, secondary or peripheral *repletiones* of this kind may still be in evidence, and in every case it is advisable (or it may be necessary) to disperse or break up these accumulations. If the source of the disorder is a discrete, readily separable foreign substance (and the disorder itself is highly acute), then the administration of an emetic is in order. In the case of a *repletio,* the procedure is somewhat more complex, since the *repletio* will be localized in a well-defined and very small area, which must be targeted with a great deal of precision, prudence, and restraint. Acupuncture may be extremely useful in this respect, but if the disorder in question is at all likely to recur (because of some congenital predisposition or some unalterable factor in the patient's life-style or environment), then drug therapy alone will be of lasting benefit. *Repletio* symptoms may range in severity from trivial to life-threatening, beginning with various symptoms associated with an excessive secretion of mucus (*pituita* symptoms) and including the formation of swellings and callosities, hemorrhaging, the appearance of ulcerations and benign growths (neoplasms), and even carcinomas. Painful localized disorders such as nonspecific neuralgia and rheumatism are also associated with *repletiones,* as are a number of different digestive disorders (which may be the direct result of improper diet or climatic changes) and recurrent, painful conditions such as migraine.

FOR PURPOSES OF COMPARISON

The foregoing discussion of the eight traditional therapeutic methods provides us with another illustration of the very different ways in which Western and Chinese medicine are accustomed to treat both the illness and the patient himself. (Among the minor disorders that are treated with *sudatio,* for example, we might mention the innumerable variants of the common cold.) Western medicine defines an illness in terms of external factors, foremost among them being an almost innumerable host of viruses and bacteria, whereas Chinese medicine is exclusively concerned with functional disturbances as a means of defining and classifying illnesses. This seems entirely fitting, since, for all the subtlety of its diagnostic technique, Chinese medicine still manages to get along with just a handful of diagnostic images—clinical pictures of separate "diseases"—and a comparable number of basic therapeutic strategies. In Western medicine, the patient becomes a battleground between the viral or bacterial invaders and the chemical countermeasures devised by the pharmaceutical industry; the patient's powers of resistance play only a subordinate role in determining the outcome of the struggle. (And when the struggle is actually waged outside the arena of the patient's body, we call it by a different name—*hygiene, preventive medicine,* or *public health.*) Since resistant viral and bacterial strains are constantly appearing on the scene, Western medicine is constantly obliged to devise fresh counter-measures to deal with them. At the same time, this is one reason why retrospective laboratory tests have become so expensive, since doctors are compelled to dispense with ordinary practical and preventive treatment and to rely on the "scattershot" method—treating the patient with wide-spectrum antibiotics but without the benefit of a comprehensive diagnosis. Here we can reduce the difference between Western and Chinese medicine to a simple antinomy—killing microbes versus supporting the patient's vital functions.

PRACTICAL PHARMACOTHERAPY: COPING WITH THE FLU

Simply to list and discuss the principal characteristics of all the traditional Chinese remedies would easily fill a volume as large as this one,[2] but without allowing ourselves to be beguiled too much by particulars, we would like to try to give some idea of how Chinese pharmacotherapy would be put into practice in a typical case—let us say a case of the flu.

Inflammation and fever are considered to be *calor* symptoms, in Western as well as Chinese medicine, but this is by no means to imply that the appearance of these symptoms in themselves justifies an immediate diagnosis of *calor*. Even for an everyday sort of ailment like the flu, Chinese medicine distinguishes at least a dozen separate diagnostic findings, so that naturally there are at least as many basic remedies whose purpose is to make these disorders disappear as quickly and unceremoniously as they came.[3] We all know that there are some varieties of the flu that are not actually accompanied by a high fever as such but by an abnormal sensitivity to temperature—the patient may shiver, he may be extremely sensitive to drafts, or he may complain that

216   a closed room is overheated and stuffy. But these individual symptoms cannot be treated directly and schematically; instead, a real diagnosis must be sought that will uncover the underlying factors that are bringing them about—and that can be treated.

Let us assume that most people who get the flu are otherwise fairly healthy, by and large, with no chronic instability in the relevant functional regions (the circle of the lungs and the airway). This means that the flu may be classified as an acute illness, recent in origin, which begins by affecting the *species* region. This may be readily confirmed by examining the patient's pulse (which will be strong but superficial) and tongue (bright red with a white coating). Now the doctor will begin treatment by administering a remedy that helps to "open up" the superficial regions of the body (*medicamenta liberantia speciei*), an ample dose of which will cause the patient to perspire freely but that in a weaker dosage will simply ensure a normal transpiration of moisture through the pores.

This should get the healing process under way, but the doctor's primary task is still to identify the prevailing direction (the vectorial resultant, to revert to the terms of our original discussion of this concept) of the heteropathy that is ultimately responsible for all these disturbances. The question is not at this point what sort of climatic or atmospheric conditions (or what currently prevalent virus) might have given rise to these symptoms, or how many additional or idiosyncratic symptoms can be identified, but rather which functional region has been pushed out of equilibrium, in what direction, and to what extent—all of the diagnostic variables that can be expressed by the single word *heteropathy*.

Thus it is possible that when all the patient's symptoms have been evaluated, an illness that is accompanied by a fever will turn out to be a manifestation of an *algor* ("cold") heteropathy—or another illness that presents similar symptoms but that has unmistakably been contracted during cold weather will turn out to be a manifestation of a *calor* heteropathy. For example, the symptoms associated with a diagnosis of *algor* may include the following: severe chills but only a moderate fever, headache, stiff neck, nonlocalized body aches, superficial but not greatly accelerated pulse, surface of the tongue extremely slick or slippery, and whitish coating on the tongue (which may build up very rapidly, depending on the gravity of the illness). These are the corresponding *calor* symptoms: unmistakably high fever, chills less pronounced (or possibly absent altogether), headache (but without the body aches), and redness around the eyes (which may also be bloodshot). The *calor* patient

(unlike the *algor* patient) will be very thirsty, his pulse both superficial
and accelerated. The tongue will be rather dry, the coating not especially
thick, with a barely detectable yellowish tinge. And, as we have seen,
these two disorders are brought about by diametrically opposite factors
(in spite of the fact that their symptoms are rather similar) and thus must
be treated by quite different means. This is why, for example, the
pharmacological category of "superficial" remedies (*medicamenta superficialia*) is further subdivided, so that a febrile *algor* heteropathy will be
treated with a "warm-superficial" remedy, a *calor* heteropathy with a
"cold-heteropathy" remedy.

Warm remedies that serve to "open up" or "free" the *species* region
when an *algor* heteropathy is present include a number of herbs of the
genus *Ephedra* (one of the few traditional Chinese remedies that has
found its way into the Western pharmacopoeia in modern times, though
its indications—the circumstances under which its use is recommended—are quite different and relatively crude and nonspecific) as well
as the twigs of the cassia tree, or Chinese cinnamon (there are at least
three varieties of Chinese cinnamon, though none of them is the source
of the familiar kitchen spice, which also plays an important role in
Chinese pharmacology); the leaves, stalks, and flowers of several different
herbs of the mint family (Labiatae), specifically of the genera *Schizonep-
tae* and *Perilla;* the roots and rhizomes of various plants of the family
Umbelliferae, specifically of the genera *Notopterygii, Ledebouriella,* and
Angelica (*Angelica dahurica* and *Angelica anomala*—the related *Angelica
sinensis* is an important medicinal plant that falls into a different
category); a variety of lovage (*Ligustica sinensis*); the root of the wild
ginger (*Asarum*) as well as the more familiar variety; and the dried
flowers of the magnolia. All of these remedies are classified as warm and
sharp, and a great many of them have a marked affinity for the function
circles of the lungs, the spleen and the stomach, the liver, and the
kidneys, so that their optimal application will naturally depend on the
diagnosis in a particular case.

And since the illness that we simply call the flu may also on closer
investigation turn out to be the result of an acute, recently developed
calor heteropathy, then the application of a cool remedy will accordingly
be necessary to open up the *species* region. A large number of herbal
remedies are also available for this purpose, including another variety of
mint (*Mentha arrensis*); mulberry leaves; chrysanthemum flowers; a
special medicinal preparation of dried, fermented (or sprouted) soybeans;
the root of the kudzu vine (genus *Pueraria*) and of a herb called

218   bupleurum (another member of the family Umbelliferae); the root of another herb, cimicifuga (less formally known as bugbane); the horsetail (genus *Equisetum*); the seeds of a member of the burdock family, *Arctium lappa;* and finally a preparation that is not really a herbal remedy at all, since it is made from the ground-up cocoons of the cicada *Cryptotympana pustulata.* All of these are classified as sharp (though less so than the corresponding *algor* remedies); the mulberry and the chrysanthemum have a bitter and a sweet *sapor* as well. The remedies in this group have an affinity for the function circles of the lungs, though, once again, this is less pronounced than in the case of the *algor* remedies.

GINGER: MILD WARMTH

Since fresh ginger is now widely available in markets (and Chinese drugstores) in Western countries, and since it plays an especially versatile role in Chinese pharmacology, we would like to say an extra word or two about it here. In Chinese drugstores, ginger root is sold fresh, dried, or roasted (candied or crystallized ginger is not used in Chinese medicine), and in each of these forms it has somewhat different effects and medicinal indications. One thing they all have in common is a distinctively sharp *sapor* and an "opening up" or "loosening" effect, insofar as they serve to mobilize the body's reserves of *qi.* Fresh ginger is regarded as mildly warm, dried ginger as warm, and roasted ginger as hot, so that the latter two may be employed as *medicamenta tepefacienta* in cases where an *algor* heteropathy of the *intima* region has been diagnosed. Ginger is very frequently prescribed on other occasions as well, primarily because it has a special affinity for those function circles whose activities are disrupted by external stress and irregular living habits—the circle of the lungs, namely, and the circles of the spleen and stomach. Ginger strengthens the organism's capacity to assimilate and to integrate external stimuli (including the effects of certain foods).

Ginger is also widely dispensed in concentrated form as the mildest of the common specifics against nausea (*inhibentia vomitus*), which means that it is generally included in any prescription for a digestive disorder of any kind or any disorder that is accompanied by loss of appetite or queasiness. (Bear in mind that about 80 percent of all therapeutic procedures in Chinese medicine involve the administration of herbal or other remedies, the vast majority of which are taken orally and absorbed through the digestive tract in the form of pills, powders, and decoctions. Ointments, salves, and suppositories are also not unknown, of course, but these are much less frequently used, since they are slower-acting and

somewhat more difficult to administer.) Ginger is also modestly effective
as an antitussive (cough remedy) and as an expectorant and is used in‑
folk medicine as well as in classical, scientific medicine—and, of course,
in Chinese cooking as well; one of the main reasons why Chinese meals,
which are extremely rich and generally eaten late in the evening, are so
easily digestible is the discreet but indispensable presence of ginger.

GINSENG: DEFENSIVE POWER

Ginseng is first mentioned in the classic pharmaceutical treatise known
as the *Bencaojing,* which dates back to the beginnings of systematic
medicine in China. Ginseng is called *renshen* in Chinese; *shen* refers to a
wide variety of medicinal roots, and *ren* simply means "man," so that
renshen means something like "the medicinal root that is shaped like a
man." Its botanical name is *Panax schinseng* C. A. Meyer, and it is a
member of the family *Aralaceae;* it grows best in the cool, moist, coastal
regions of the temperate zone, which means that it is largely confined to
a few small areas in Korea and the adjacent districts of eastern
Manchuria. (A similar species is native to the Pacific Northwest Coast of
North America). It takes between six and eight years before the root has
reached full size and is ready to be harvested; by that time it has assumed
the proportions of a full-grown homunculus, with head and trunk, arms
and legs in place. Ginseng has always been scarce in the wild state in
China and priced accordingly; since the eighteenth century a herb of the
family Campanulaceae called *Codonopsis tangshen* Oliver has been widely
employed as a substitute, since it has many, though not all, of the
important medicinal properties of ginseng and is cultivated today as far
south as central China.

We hasten to point out, by the way, that ginseng has never been
regarded as a panacea in Chinese folk medicine (let alone in scientific
medicine) and has never been thought to confer immortality or even to
prolong life (except in the way that any medicinal substance may be
thought to do so). Chinese folk medicine, and especially Taoism in its
magical and alchemical aspect, have indeed come up with a number of
elixirs of long life; apart from certain alchemical concoctions that
contained mercury amalgam, most of these were derived from mush‑
rooms of the genus *Ganoderma,* which in recent years have been the
object of rigorous pharmacological investigation (this time conducted
according to Western scientific criteria). Ginseng, however, has never
enjoyed such a reputation in East Asia.

Ginseng is classified with the *medicamenta supplentia qi,* remedies that

220 help to replenish or, in this case, enhance the potential for active release of the body's reserves of energy. More precisely, ginseng root completes the potentiation of *qi primum,* innate active energy. Because of its sweet, slightly bitter *sapor,* it works directly on the function circles of the spleen and stomach and the circle of the lungs. "Ginseng conducts energy to the circles of the spleen and the lungs. It triggers the production of active fluids, and it has a calming effect." The circle of the spleen corresponds to the transformation phase of earth and acts as the "mediator," presiding over the process of integration, i.e., the process of assimilating external energy and transforming it into one's own. This circle is accordingly regarded as the central reservoir of *qi ascitum,* "acquired constitutional energy," thought also to be the source or the medium of all our learned or acquired behavior, with the emphasis on the customary or the habitual (including bad habits, to be sure). A deficiency in this circle thus affects much more than the soundness of the individual's digestion, since he can no longer replace the energy he has expended by means of the normal process of assimilating energy (or sensory impressions) from the outside world.

The circle of the lungs regulates the rhythm of all our activities and ensures that physiological energy is uniformly distributed throughout the body. The *perfectio,* the consummate somatic embodiment or representation of this circle is the skin, the source of the body's defensive energy. Thus these two circles may be regarded as the body's primary defense against all harmful substances or stimuli, and both circles are strengthened and stabilized by the effects of ginseng. Specifically, the administration of ginseng root is indicated for *inanitas qi,* as evidenced by a frail or disappearing pulse; weak, shallow, and raspy breathing; continuous perspiration; a feeling of coldness in the extremities (all of which may follow a severe loss of blood or other bodily fluids); *inanitas* of the circle of the lungs, the symptoms of which include soft, even breathing that becomes irregular after the slightest exertion, as well as fatigue and lack of stamina; and *inanitas* of the circle of the spleen, the symptoms of which include weakness and exhaustion, loss of appetite and a feeling of tension in the abdominal region. A Chinese doctor will always prescribe ginseng in combination with some other remedy, which, depending on the individual diagnosis, will either operate in the same direction (such as the rhizome of the herb *Atractylodis*) or in the opposite direction (a mushroom of the genus *Poria*), even though the disorders just mentioned will generally respond to treatment with ginseng alone. (This last statement is subject to the caveat that certain of the *individual symptoms*

mentioned earlier may not be the result of an *inanitas* at all; e.g., if a   221
patient who is found to be suffering from fatigue or exhaustion also
exhibits loud, stertorous breathing and a moving pulse, then a dose of
ginseng will only serve to aggravate this condition.)

Chinese druggists, like all Chinese merchants, have always obeyed the
maxim that it is bad business to try to force anything on a customer that
he doesn't really need (while acknowledging, of course, that the customer
may require some guidance in determining what his real needs are). In
imperial times it was observed that the privileged classes—mandarins
and particularly their wives and the older members of their households—
very often complained of a kind of lassitude or enervated state brought
on by a sedentary mode of life and a surfeit of rich food. Druggists would
entice these prosperous *inanitas* patients with phrases like "Now the age
of austerity [i.e., middle age] is knocking at the door. Shield yourself
from its cruelest blows—dose yourself with our *supplentia* and win back
your depleted vigor!" So much the better, of course, that the most
versatile of these *supplentia* was also the costliest and hardest to come by.
Today ginseng is widely available, no longer beyond the reach of the
ordinary worker or peasant, but there has never been much of a vogue
for it, as there has in the West in recent years, nor could it be considered
a staple household remedy. (Only the credulous and simpleminded
foreign devils would actually believe that a daily decoction of ginseng
could restore lost virility as well as vitality and is thus indispensable to
every man who hopes to remain vigorous through "the age of austerity.")

External Therapy: Acupuncture and Moxa

THE Chinese themselves are in part responsible for the widespread Western notion that acupuncture is strictly a hit-or-miss, or empirical, proposition. As we have pointed out, the practice of acupuncture has never been limited to licensed professionals in China (any more than, say, the management of a massage parlor or a gymnasium has been restricted to board-certified physicians in the West). Moreover, the vast majority of acupuncturists in East Asia have had only the sketchiest introduction to the theoretical foundations of acu-moxa-therapy (this often includes the classical diagnostic techniques as well)—whether they be state-trained "barefoot doctors," old-style professionals who have learned the craft (rather than the science) from a teacher, or physicians whose background is primarily in Western medicine. (In this respect they might be likened to truck drivers who have simply learned how to drive their trucks and have scarcely a clue as to how the carburetor or the differential works.) However, there is one important difference between the East Asian practitioners of this rudimentary form of acu-moxa-therapy and their European and North American counterparts: In China, the practice of the *technique* of acupuncture is so widespread that almost every Chinese can tell immediately whether he has entrusted himself to the hands of an expert or a quack.

What is more, the Chinese are generally aware of what acupuncture can and cannot be expected to accomplish. It is simply a technique by means of which a surplus of energy can be dislodged from the arterial pathways, or an obstructive or congestive accumulation of energy can be dissipated, or a localized excess accumulation of energy can be diverted to relieve a localized deficiency. Moxibustion—therapeutic combustion of a herb called mugwort (*Artemisia vulgaris*) on the skin above an impulse point—may similarly be regarded as a technique of *suppletio*, of inducing an influx of energy into a particular region (further provided

224   that this redirected flow of energy is strictly temporary and always of active polarity). Clearly in cases where this procedure seems appropriate in light of a specific diagnosis—when the therapeutic technique corresponds to the diagnostic findings as neatly as the key fits the lock—then the therapy may be reasonably expected to be successful. In cases where such a diagnosis is lacking, of course, then the use of acupuncture really *is* no more than a hit-or-miss proposition and has nothing to do with science at all or even with "pure" or elegant technique. That is why the sort of treatment that passes under the name of acupuncture in the West is necessarily to be viewed with caution, and it is equally regrettable that the academic medical establishment, in concert with the medical organizations most directly involved, has chosen to give its active or tacit encouragement to this sort of dilettantism—even though acupuncturists have had their own professional associations (in Europe at least) for almost fifty years and a small handful of doctors have consistently been lobbying for a higher standard of instruction, if only in the technical aspects of the discipline.

With respect to this latter point, a duly constituted scientific commission—albeit one whose members, for the most part, had never witnessed an acupuncture session or treated a patient by this means and none of whom had so much as a nodding acquaintance with the basic theoretical principles involved—recently delivered itself of the following official pronouncement: "Acupuncture is a procedure whose basic scientific foundations have yet to be explained. Accordingly, this question [of establishing guidelines for its use, technical standards, etc.] should be left to the individual practitioner." In other words, since acupuncture is ostensibly a form of therapy with no proven scientific or theoretical basis, then the question of establishing such professional standards is moot, and anyone (i.e., any doctor) who wants to set himself up in practice as an acupuncturist may legitimately do so without bothering about formalities. Even academic medicine, which had previously extended a reluctantly outstretched hand in the general direction of therapeutic acupuncture, has not only neglected to provide but also has explicitly repudiated the need for any formal, rational foundation for its experiments with acupuncture and has thus far preferred to keep things on a strictly pragmatic basis.

BRIEF TECHNICAL DIGRESSION

We feel that such a digression is justified by the current state of the literature on acupuncture available in the West, which sometimes conveys a fairly fantastic impression of what therapeutic acupuncture really involves. To begin with, there is the question of selecting and locating the appropriate impulse points. The stock image from the Sunday supplement picture file on acupuncture generally has the patient stuck full of needles like a hedgehog, but in fact the treatment of a functional disorder requires that only between one and four or five needles be inserted at the same time. Anyone who has been treated with acupuncture, whether by an expert or a practitioner of more modest competence, can testify that a single needle inserted out of place, or a single needle too many, can easily impair or even counteract the effects of the needles that have been placed correctly.

For many years now, acupuncture atlases and wall charts have been available to assist the practitioner in locating the correct impulse points; anyone who has ever visited an acupuncturist's office will be familiar at least with the latter, which generally presents a series of views of the interior of the body, showing the skeleton and internal organs, nervous and vascular systems as the background for a schematic representation of the arterial pathways and the impulse points. Nowadays the acupuncturists may also use an electronic sensor about the size of a ballpoint pen with a probe at the tip, and an attached handgrip (of opposite polarity) that is held by the patient. A weak electric current that can be increased at will flows through the sensor and the handgrip; the basic principle involved is that acupuncture points have been found to evince a highly variable resistance to an electric current as compared with the surrounding tissue. Though significant technical improvements have been made in recent years, the accuracy of the sensor cannot be relied on absolutely; it may be deceived by local fluctuations in electroconductivity caused by differing amounts of moisture on the skin or by a film of grease or oil, whether natural or artificial, on the skin surface. The sensor is thus not quite equal to the task in itself, but it remains a useful auxiliary device.

For the past two thousand years, Chinese acupuncturists have been able to locate the impulse points exactly by probing with their fingers and applying their detailed knowledge of the body's normal proportions. An old-fashioned acupuncture chart that lacks the realistic background detail described above may seem remarkably primitive to us today, but traditional practitioners never had much difficulty finding what they were looking for. These charts were intended only to show the relative positions of the pathways and the relative distances between consecutive impulse points; anatomical details were included only as useful landmarks or orientation points—e.g., to indicate that a given pathway (as

226   extrapolated from a sequence of points) passes between a fold or a wrinkle in the skin and a bony process or projection. When the acupuncturist follows along this line with his fingers, he will be able to recognize the individual impulse point by touch; a great many of them (most of those on the back, the extremities, and the joints) feel like actual depressions in the skin with elastic boundaries or, more rarely, like callosities (hard patches) in an otherwise perfectly smooth and flexible surface. This is especially likely to be the case when the function that activates a pathway is at all volatile or erratic (*shidong* is the Chinese term for this, meaning that it "moves around"). The patient may also be aware of their location as well, since certain functional disorders may be accompanied by a heightened sensitivity in the corresponding impulse points, particularly in the case of the *inductoria dorsalia* (see page 127) as well as various other points that may be affected by *repletio* heteropathies and, by definition, the *foramina ad hoc* (see page 123).

There are still a number of points that cannot be located directly by palpation and in which the patient need not necessarily experience a heightened sensitivity to pressure. Some of these are found on the extremities, most on the ventral (front) side of the body and on the abdomen in particular (as well as a number of points on the head and face that may be stimulated as part of a special therapeutic procedure). These points can be located only by measurement, though not by simple linear measurement, as with a tape measure; instead, their locations must be determined indirectly, on the basis of bionomic ratios derived from the patient's known bodily proportions. Thus the acupuncturist may deduce that a given point is to be found at a given distance from an unambiguous anatomical reference point, such as a bony projection. When the point in question is on the head or face, the acupuncturist may use a grease pencil and measuring cord, rather in the manner of a surveyor, to mark off its location.

As for the needles themselves, a Chinese acupuncturist invariably uses steel needles (nowadays made out of high-grade surgical steel), which are available in various lengths and diameters. The size most frequently used is about a quarter of a millimeter in diameter and from an inch to an inch and a half long (about 2.5–4 cm), not including the handgrip. Others range in length between about half an inch to as much as a foot. The manner in which the needle is to be inserted has been determined *for each individual point* on the basis of two thousand years' clinical experience. The depth of the insertion, for example, may vary from a

fraction of a millimeter to about ten centimeters, the average depth being
about one or two centimeters.

According to the classical Chinese technique, the needle is held
between thumb and forefinger of the right hand and guided by the
thumb and forefinger of the left hand, held over the point of insertion.
The angle of insertion may be level or oblique, the motion slow and
delicate or brisk and instantaneous, according to the therapeutic goals of
the treatment. The acupuncturist must have a sure and practiced touch
to be able to "feel" the characteristic resistance of the tissue (and to make
sure the needle has been inserted to the proper depth), and, of course, the
patient himself may be of some assistance in this respect. With the
exception of a few problematical areas (the fingers and toes, the soles of
the feet), a needle may be painlessly inserted to whatever depth is
required (e.g., in the joints or the abdominal region). If the needle has
been correctly positioned, the patient begins to feel the "energy of
encounter" (*de qi*), a sensation that is not really painful and is experienced
by some people as rather pleasant. This sensation is often accompanied
by a spontaneous alleviation of symptoms after the needle has remained
in place for five or ten minutes, at which point it may make sense for the
therapist to remove and replace the needle to recapture this sensation. As
a rule, however, the needle remains in place from fifteen to thirty
minutes and is then either painlessly withdrawn or falls out of its own
accord.

The widespread use of therapeutic acupuncture in the West, both by
physicians and lay practitioners, has helped to relieve the suffering of
many thousands of patients since its advent in the early 1970s, but it has
also touched off a certain amount of controversy and even provoked an
occasional strident suggestion to the effect that acupuncture should either
be banned outright or strictly reserved for the use of licensed physicians.
Such protests have appeared in publications for the general reader as well
as professional journals, and the argument for this point of view
generally rests on the assumption that acupuncture is no more than
mesmerism in modern dress, that it relies entirely on the power of
suggestion, and, less controversially, that it is unadvisable to have
unqualified practitioners sticking needles into people, which introduces
the risk of injury or infection and perhaps even death.

As to this first point, anyone who has even the slightest familiarity
with the rational, theoretical system underlying the practice of Chinese
medicine—or who has become convinced by examining the relevant

228   clinical data or by direct experience of the close correlation between the theoretically predictable and the actual outcome of a given procedure—does not have to be told that acupuncture has been shown to have prompt and precise effects on unconscious patients (and household pets, for that matter) in order to discard this argument out of hand. As for the problem of injury or infection, no one will deny that the irresponsible use of acupuncture needles could indeed cause serious injury. But anyone who tries to make a case for a total or partial ban on acupuncture—whether on the basis of the potential hazards involved or of actual reported cases of malpractice or clinical mishap—should bear in mind that here in the West it is left entirely up to private initiative to compensate for the deficiencies of academic medicine in this respect. In other words, anyone who practices acupuncture will most probably be self-taught (or taught by someone who has supplemented his own casual mastery of the subject with a few years of self-supervised experimentation). Anyone who has had the opportunity to observe a large number of acupuncturists at work over the years may well become less concerned with the risk of accidental injury than with the far greater likelihood that treatment will be completely ineffective—when the acupuncturist inserts a needle inaccurately or superficially, or removes it almost immediately after insertion. Others rely chiefly on such hybrid forms of therapy as laser acupuncture, auriculotherapy, and acupressure, and although of course a successful treatment is not to be ruled out unconditionally, none of these really has any claim to the high level of predictability and reliability associated with classical acupuncture therapy.

MOXIBUSTION

The traditional, and in East Asia the most invariable, complement to acupuncture therapy is moxibustion, and, as we have mentioned, these two therapeutic techniques are generally referred to collectively as *zhenjiu,* acu-moxa-therapy. The treatment begins with the therapist forming the dried mugwort leaves into a ball with his fingers; the smallest of the three customary sizes is scarcely bigger than a grain of wheat, at most, and is placed directly over the impulse point with a pair of tweezers and ignited with the glowing tip of a stick of incense. The moxa is totally consumed within a fraction of a second, and the treatment may be repeated several times in the same spot without burning the skin. A somewhat larger ball, about the size of a pea, may leave a small reddish patch on the skin, but a single treatment will never leave a burn. A still larger ball, about the size of a cherry, is almost never applied to the skin directly; generally a slice of fresh ginger or garlic (or in the case of certain impulse points in the vicinity of the navel, a small heap of salt) is interposed to provide insulation. The moxa is ignited in a candle flame and set in place with a pair of tweezers or chopsticks. The moxa is removed as soon as the patient reports that he can feel the heat of the flame, often before the moxa has been totally consumed. Larger balls of moxa may be applied directly to the skin on occasion, with the express purpose of producing a burn (a procedure that seems comparable to the obsolete Western medical practice of cauterization), but in all other cases the sole purpose of moxa therapy is to stimulate the impulse points with intermittent but fairly intense heat. Traditional Chinese medical texts invariably specify whether a given point is to be stimulated with acupuncture, with moxa (and in what amount), or both.

NONTRADITIONAL VARIANTS: ACUANALGESIA

A great many doctors (and patients) profess to see no difference between classical acupuncture therapy and *acuanalgesia* (*zhenci masui*), the use of acupuncture needles to produce an analgesic (pain-suppressing) or an anesthetic effect. The main thing these two procedures have in common is that needles are employed in each case, and they differ considerably in that the impulse points are stimulated to an almost incomparably greater degree in acuanalgesia and in that the process of selecting the points to be stimulated in acuanalgesia has come to rely less and less on traditional Chinese foraminology (so that eventually there may appear to be absolutely no connection whatever with classical theory or practice). When acuanalgesia was first developed in China, the needle was continuously rotated by hand or applied with an up-and-down motion like that of a sewing machine. Electrostimulation was introduced shortly after that, with either a weak or a frequently-modulated direct current of a given voltage flowing through the needle. (Even so, the intensity of the stimulus may be as much as a hundred thousand times as great as in traditional acupuncture.)

At first the current was applied to the familiar *foramina* of classical medicine, though these were chosen not because of their affinity for a particular function circle but simply because of their location with respect to a certain area of the body. Though this was not exactly the intention of these early experiments, later developments in acuanesthesia (due to the impetus of both Western and Chinese doctors who were involved) gradually began to shift the theoretical foundations of the discipline, so that today it is exclusively based on a compartmentalized

230   Western neurological model. Today, in the West as well as in China, major operations, such as the removal or resection of an organ, heart surgery, and brain surgery, are carried out with the help of acuanesthesia, though usually in combination with more conventional chemical anesthetics. In such cases the intensity of the electrical stimulation is literally almost as much as the patient can bear—perhaps only to be likened to the stimulus of a conventional acupuncture needle in the way that the buzzing of a honeybee may be compared to the throbbing of a jackhammer. From the standpoint of traditional Chinese medicine, such a procedure would be regarded as both unspecific and overwhelming; the therapeutic stimulus of an acupuncture needle produces almost no measurable functional change—the results are only barely perceptible by the patient, whereas the level of stimulation involved in acuanalgesia simply overloads or shuts down a large portion of the patient's sensory apparatus. Accordingly, it seems only appropriate that further technical and conceptual developments in acuanalgesia should be sought within the realm of Western neurology rather than traditional Chinese medicine.

AURICULOTHERAPY

Classical foraminology recognizes only four impulse points on cardinal pathways in or in the vicinity of the ears—hardly enough to provide a basis for a self-contained, comprehensive therapeutic system, or so it would appear. Nevertheless, in 1958 French physician Paul Nogier began to identify a series of unambiguous functional connections between various parts of the external ear and certain organs or organ systems; this enabled him to establish a complete mapping of these auricular reflex zones, as he called them, onto their somatic counterparts. Accounts of Nogier's discovery began to appear in China within a year or two after they were published in the *Deutsche Zeitschrift für Akupunktur,* and Nogier's technique of treating organic disorders by inserting acupuncture needles into the muscle of the ear was firmly established within a few more years as a respectable offshoot of traditional acupuncture therapy.

Nogier was obliged to develop his own diagnostic methods, since, for example, the reflex zones and points on the external ear are too small and too close together to be located with the fingers (though the electronic sensor is more reliable here than elsewhere, since the moisture level and thus the electroconductivity of the skin are relatively uniform). It is certainly not to its discredit that in the first twenty-five years of its

existence auriculotherapy has not attained the same level of systemization
and clinical refinement as classical acupuncture. In fact, auriculotherapy
has been widely adopted as a standard clinical technique in East Asia,
and a number of Asian researchers[4] have become convinced that
auriculotherapy may prove to be a more flexible therapeutic instrument
in dealing with certain acute organic disorders than classical acupuncture.
Certainly the fact that auriculotherapy was developed under the aegis of
Western theoretical medicine would tend to facilitate its acceptance as a
reputable clinical procedure.

ELECTROACUPUNCTURE

Electroacupuncture, in direct contrast to auriculotherapy, is a combination of Western technique and Chinese theoretical postulates. After the
Second World War, experiments were carried out in Japan, Korea, West
Germany, and the Soviet Union attempting to measure the electric
potential at specific impulse points and to stimulate these points with an
electric current flowing through an electrode or a conventional acupuncture needle. Mass-produced "acupuncture boxes" first came onto the
market in the late 1950s, in the People's Republic of China and
elsewhere. This alliance of precise diagnostic method with Western
precision electronics might appear to be quite promising at first glance,
but thus far the clinical results achieved by electroacupuncture have been
very disappointing.

There are two main reasons for this. The first is the methodologically
slipshod and overly eclectic approach adopted by the proponents of this
technique. They have failed to take into account the radical differences
between the Chinese concept of a function circle and the Western
concept of an organ, and they have persistently tried to gloss over this
crucial distinction in their interpretation of empirical data. The second
reason is one we have already alluded to—the practical difficulties
involved in developing an electronic monitoring device that can cope
with the subtleties of Chinese diagnosis. At the moment it seems that a
highly experienced specialist in electroacupuncture might be able to get
respectable empirical results by this means but that the majority of
practicing physicians would be hard pressed to do so within a tolerable
degree of accuracy.

LASERACUPUNCTURE

For the past decade compact and efficient devices have been available
that can focus a beam of laser light (usually toward the red end of the

232   spectrum) of controlled intensity on an individual impulse point. It cannot be denied that a technique of this kind, which cannot harm the patient and is free from potential mechanical defects, is greatly desirable in principle. Here, too, the question remains, however, whether the effects of stimulating an impulse point with laser light are really comparable to those of the much more complex procedure of inserting an acupuncture needle to the same (or to a much greater) depth. As much as we might applaud the news that experiments along these lines are to be continued, for the present it is far from certain that such a procedure (even in any foreseeable future state of the art) will have anything to contribute to the discipline of classical acupuncture.

ACUPRESSURE

This involves the localized stimulation of impulse points with the fingertips, a pencil, or a specially designed blunt stylus. As far as we know, acupressure was originally developed by masseurs in the Orient (in Japan primarily) during the early years of this century; it has recently come to enjoy considerable popularity in Europe and North America as well (frequently under its Japanese name, *shiatsu*). Anyone who is familiar with acupressure can attest to the fact that it can indeed bring relief from temporary, superficial discomfort, such as a headache brought about by a sudden change in the weather, an acutely stopped-up nose, or a mild digestive disorder. Though clearly inspired by the example of classical acupuncture, acupressure should accordingly be regarded more as a kind of sophisticated home remedy (which is more or less what its inventors intended it to be) than a full-fledged medical treatment.

VII

THE HISTORY OF CHINESE MEDICINE

The Rediscovery of Classical Medical Science in China

A YOUNG worker named Liu Wenzhang was smiling as he lay on the operating table in the Workers', Soldiers', and Peasants' Hospital in Shanghai. As the doctors were cutting away a section of his skull preparatory to removing a brain tumor, he continued to carry on a conversation with his sister, explaining to onlookers, "I feel fine. I just have a little pain in the top of my head and in my belly, and I'm kind of tired." While his sister held a cup of cool water to his lips, the chief surgeon told him, "We're going in through the top of your head now, Comrade Liu, but you've got absolutely nothing to worry about." The operation began at 9:15 A.M. First the anesthetist inserted five thin needles into Liu's left ear; there was no need for any other anesthetic. Liu remained fully conscious throughout the entire four-and-a-half-hour operation, one of the most grueling procedures in the repertory of modern surgery. After the operation was over, the surgeons tested Liu's reactions and announced, "He's doing fine. There's been no impairment of any vital functions, and the bleeding is under control."[1]

The removal of Comrade Liu's tumor in this manner was the eventual result of Chairman Mao's public-health policy, as adumbrated during the struggle against the Japanese and as definitively set forth in this communiqué of 1958: "Chinese medicine and pharmacology are a vast treasure trove. We should make every effort to investigate them further and to raise them to a higher level of development."[2] The chairman's predilection for traditional medicine, which can be traced as far back as the era of the Long March, was originally hedged with reservations and at all times strictly pragmatic. In 1944, when his forces were still heavily engaged against the Japanese, he wrote: "In the Shaanxi-Gansu-Ninyxia region [in the Northwest], out of a population of a million and a half there are still a million illiterates and two thousand herb doctors. . . . The death rate is very high. Under these conditions if we were to rely solely

236   and exclusively on modern doctors, then we would not be able to accomplish anything. Modern doctors are naturally to be preferred to the old-fashioned sort, but when the modern doctors are indifferent to the sufferings of the people, when they refuse to train medical personnel to serve the people, when they refuse to join forces with the more than one thousand herb doctors who are already on hand in the frontier regions, then in reality it is only the herb doctors they are helping by this behavior, rather than themselves."[3]

Mao's public-health policy began with the idea of mobilizing all available material and intellectual resources—whether "modern" or "old-fashioned" in their orientation—against the various plagues and infectious scourges by which the Chinese people were afflicted in wartime and, in general, to minister to the basic medical needs of the "broad masses of the people." One doctor who was both a historian and an architect of this policy was an American, George Hatem, who had first arrived in Shanghai in 1933 "to study some tropical medicine." Instead he found himself treating patients who were on the edge of starvation, who had no money to spare for doctors or drugs. He decided to stay on in China and made contact with Mao's army early in the course of the Long March. Taking the *nom de guerre* of "Dr. Ma Hai-teh," he embarked on a campaign to eradicate elephantiasis, leprosy, bubonic plague, malaria, and a number of other endemic diseases from the "liberated area" of North China; he later recalled that he had set out after the syphilis spirochete "and chased it back across the steppes of Inner Mongolia."

According to Dr. Hatem, the astonishingly rapid success of Mao's public-health policy could be attributed primarily to the systematic recruitment of barefoot doctors, the encouragement of traditional medicine, and the establishment of a cooperative health insurance scheme that brought decent medical care within the reach of the urban proletariat for the first time in recent history. Of all these factors, the first was perhaps the most crucial: "The provision of medical services to the grass roots—the constant day-to-day availability that works year in and year out, that continuing drip-drop that brings the steady results. The campaigns are more dramatic, but it is the day-to-day follow-through work that results in the eradication of disease. This was in addition to keeping a tab on the general state of health in the whole population. People are very healthy now. They get a good start through proper nourishment, infant care, and more generalized knowledge of how to look after children, so that you get a healthier youth growing up from the start. But the secret of the glowing health that visitors remark on in the street is this constant day in, day out availability of health care. People know the service is there—and they use it."[4]

Although the major thrust of Mao's policy was in the direction of intense personal commitment and the mobilization of basic human resources rather than technical or scientific progress, it is true that classical medical science experienced something of a renaissance during the 1950s. Academies of traditional medicine were established in all of China's major cities, beginning in 1949. And, as we have seen, the daunting task of assembling, editing, and reprinting a complete library of classical medical and pharmacological texts was undertaken in the late 1950s (though unfortunately a number of these handsome volumes are still available only in very limited editions). After several centuries of neglect (or worse), the contents of this medical treasure trove were displayed before the eyes of scholars once again, and the long, slow decline of traditional medicine was dramatically reversed in a very few years.

You may recall that traditional medicine had been marked down for extinction by the Nationalist regime not too many years earlier, and in fact the first meeting of the National Board of Health in Nanking in February 1929 had resulted in a "proposal for the suppression of indigenous curative practices." Before this proposal could be implemented, however, more than two thousand medical clinics shut their doors in protest, and outraged herb doctors from all over the nation converged on Shanghai for a mass rally on March 17. Not long after that, the decree was rescinded, partially in response to this nationwide groundswell of protest, partially because—according to British physician Joshua S. Horn, a longtime resident in China—"many prominent Kuomintang officials were themselves devotees of the darker and more mystical forms of traditional medicine."[5]

Though at that time the practice of traditional medicine was indeed in a very sorry state and hardly deserved to be called medicine at all, it still retained the patronage and confidence of almost everyone in China, whereas Western-style doctors were still regarded with some mistrust. Certainly people were well aware of the fact that the suppression of "indigenous curative practices" would have left the vast majority of the population completely bereft of medical care, and it is difficult not to agree with Horn that this episode represents "one of those futile attempts to 'modernize' China"[6] that were typical of the Kuomintang regime. However, it would be another twenty years before this policy could be

238   reversed and almost fifty years before this new impetus provided to Chinese medicine by Chairman Mao would bring it to the attention of the world.

Today we realize that a great age of technical and scientific achievement came to an end in China just as a new scientific age was about to begin in the West. (Two of the most portentous technical developments of this period—the invention of paper and printing, first from wood blocks, later from movable type—also played an important if not always constructive role in the history of Chinese medicine.) There may be a lesson for us in the two-thousand-year history of classical Chinese medicine—fifteen centuries of systematic refinement and innovation followed by five centuries of stagnation and decline, to the brink of extinction as a scientific discipline—that extends far beyond the realm of medicine or the history of science. Rather than pursue these speculations at the moment, however, we would like to work our way back to the origins of Chinese medicine and conclude our study with a brief survey of its history, in the hope of shedding additional light on the basic theoretical principles we have been discussing thus far, as well as conveying a clearer idea of the real significance of the revival of the study and practice of traditional medicine in the People's Republic of China (and elsewhere) today.

Great Doctors and the Classical Texts

NO fewer than eleven celebrated doctors of antiquity were enshrined in the traditional Chinese pantheon, and until the early years of this century tablets bearing their names were venerated in the "temple of the medicine kings" (*yaowangmiao*) and their spirits were tempted by means of sacrificial offerings to perform special feats of medical intervention. We have already encountered two of the eleven so honored, the great Bian Que and Chunyu Yi; the others are Qi Po, Leigong, Zhang Zhongjing (or Zhang Ji), Hua Tuo, Wang Shuhe, Ge Hong (known to literature as Bao Puzi), Huangfu Mi, Sun Simo, and Li Shishzhen. These temples were also dedicated to the cults of the legendary "first emperors," Shennong and Huangdi, reputed to be the founders of classical Chinese medicine as well as the authors of a number of venerable medical texts (actually the work of writers of a much later period than that in which the first emperors were said to have flourished—the third millennium B.C.—who were prepared to forgo the pleasures of literary recognition in return for securing a more respectful hearing for their books).

Shennong was also renowned as the inventor of agriculture, "the Master of Husbandry," and revered as "the Pharmacist Sage," patron of herbalists and apothecaries, who brought offerings to his shrine on the first day of the new and the full moon (at which times they also sold their wares at reduced prices). The great catalogue of remedies traditionally ascribed to Shennong, the *Shennong Bencaojing* (*Pharmaceutical Classic of the Master of Husbandry*), is the earliest work of its kind in Chinese literature; fragments of the lost original are preserved in an edition prepared by the physician Tao Honjing early in the sixth century A.D., though the text must have been substantially altered in the intervening five or six centuries of oral and scribal transmission.

Huangdi, the second of these legendary emperors, is already well

240   known to us as the Yellow Prince. The treatise on medicine that is traditionally ascribed to him, the *Huangdi Neijing* (*The Yellow Prince's Classic of Internal Medicine*), is the earliest systematic compilation of medical lore, the most frequently cited of all the classic texts, and, all in all, a work that is without parallel in the history of the natural sciences. The original text must have been composed in about the third century B.C. (since it is repeatedly mentioned in the official catalogues of scholarly works of the Han dynasty). We may assume that its authors followed the usual practice of attributing it to a legendary sage like Huangdi in the hope of vanquishing any doubts that their contemporaries might have had about this radically new scientific approach to the art of healing. In its present form the *Huangdi Neijing* consists of two main parts of exactly eighty-one chapters each; a later contributor, the medicine king Zhang Zhongjing (second century A.D.), affixed the title *Suwen* (*Elementary Questions*) to the first part. The critical edition of the *Suwen* prepared by the scholar Wang Bing in 762 was the first to be printed (perhaps a century or so later) and for many years was not only the most widely available but was also thought to be the most reliable (until a careful comparison with the manuscript sources revealed several centuries later that at least half of the text, notably a long excursus on the five transformation phases, had been concocted by Wang Bing himself as a vehicle for his own ruminations on medical science).

The second part of the *Huangdi Neijing,* which has come to be known as the *Lingshu* (*Focal Point of Constructive Force*), has an even more intricate pedigree. An early version, the *Waijing* (*Classic of External Medicine*), is mentioned in the Han dynasty catalogues but has not come down to us in its original form. In the third century A.D. the historian Huangfu Mi published an important book entitled *Zhenjiu Jiayjing* (*Systematic Classic of Needles and Moxa*), the earliest treatment of this subject whose provenance has been established with certainty. Huangfu Mi claims to have relied heavily on *The Yellow Prince's Classic* as well as another work, titled *Zhenjing* (*The Needle Classic*), and we have no reason to doubt him on this point, even though the earliest version of the *Zhenjing* that has come down to us dates back only as far as the ninth century A.D. According to the imperial archives, an ancient manuscript of the *Zhenjing* had turned up in Korea and was presented to the emperor of China; more probably this was a contemporary reconstruction of the vanished original, whose composition was accordingly backdated to lend it the cachet of a rediscovered classic. At any rate, this reconstituted "classic of external medicine," which deals primarily with acupuncture,

has been known as the *Lingshu* (*Focal Point of Constructive Force*) since
the end of the eleventh century.

Though the exact chronology of these works remains obscure (as was their authors' intention, of course), we are at least justified in concluding that all of the principal tenets of Chinese medical theory had already been incorporated into the *Suwen,* which was composed at about the same time that the scarcely less definitive *Corpus hippocraticum* appeared in the West. The theory of the function circles, the systematic mapping of the impulse points and the pathways, the diagnostic significance of the pathological agents and the *emotiones,* and the theoretical foundations of Chinese diagnostic medicine in general can all be found in its pages. The advent of the printed book in the ninth century (movable type was introduced perhaps two centuries later) had a great deal to do with the dissemination of this knowledge (albeit, as we have seen, in a highly adulterated form at first), but by now we have already gotten well ahead of our story. The origins and early development of Chinese medicine, as of many other aspects of classical Chinese culture, were heavily influenced by the tension, not to say rivalry, between two great schools of thought, Taoism and Confucianism, and this is the subject we would like to turn to next.

TAOISM

The teachings of Taoism are traditionally associated with the philosopher Laozi (Lao-tse), but Taoism as a philosophy seems to have been in existence for some time before the birth of its supposed founder (the name of the Yellow Prince occasionally crops up in this connection as well). At any rate, *The Yellow Prince's Classic* is clearly in the Taoist tradition, which emphasizes not only a harmonious relationship between man and nature but also the necessity of observing natural processes accurately and precisely (in this respect the Taoists might be thought of as the first empiricists). In this way, man can become familiar with the "rules" or the inner workings of nature, and this in turn will enable him to understand the ways in which these earthly occurrences take their place in the greater harmony of the cosmos.

You may recall a passage we quoted earlier from *The Yellow Prince's Classic* (see page 108) that occurs very near the beginning of the book and in which the Yellow Prince, "a perfectly accomplished spirit," makes his way to Heaven to ask the immortals why it was that the men of former times managed to live to the age of two hundred "without their natural vigor being in any way abated." One of the immortals, the Count of Qi,

242   explains to him that the ancients were well acquainted with the Tao, that they lived in accordance with the principles of *yin* and *yang,* and that "they sought harmony through the useful arts and sciences and the mastery of numbers." Finally, in contrast to the decadent moderns who live only for the pursuit of pleasure "and refuse to acquaint themselves with the rules of nature," the ancients were temperate in their habits "and shunned vain strivings and heedless exertions, so that like demigods, they were able to retain their bodily forms throughout the span of years that is ordained by Heaven and only forsook this earthly existence after they had reached a hundred."[7] Finally, the count explains, the inevitable result of a life of hedonism, immoderation, and heedless ignorance of the Tao is a gradual deterioration of individual orthopathy and an unnaturally shortened life-span.

In the Taoist scheme of things, individual orthopathy, good health, was regarded as an extension or a reflection of cosmic harmony and, in everyday terms, a goal that could be achieved by various different means—proper diet and the observance of certain hygienic, medical, and in later times even magical precautions. In this respect it is worth noting that though magic and the occult did eventually come to play an important role in Taoist ritual and speculative philosophy, there is absolutely no trace of this in *The Yellow Prince's Classic* (and in fact religious observances of any kind are barely mentioned). The sort of scientific medicine we are concerned with in this book was to remain almost entirely free of any kind of occultist influence, though one often gets the impression from reading Western writers' descriptions of the subject that "Chinese medicine" is inextricably entangled with mysticism, magic, and the supernatural. It should be noted that statements of this kind, when not actually prompted by prejudice or malice, are either the result of an uncritical reliance on outdated and inaccurate (usually nineteenth-century) sources or of a fundamental (though perhaps no less unoriginal) misunderstanding of the nature of Chinese medicine and Chinese science.

The way in which the classical medical texts manage to harmonize empirical observation with the Taoist view of the cosmos as an infinite series of correspondences and proportions and significant numerical ratios is illustrated by this passage from the *Suwen* in which the count presents a kind of Taoist version of the Seven Ages of Man:

THE PRINCE: When people become too old to bear or beget children, does this mean that their innate constitutional forces are exhausted, or is this the effect of some natural [numerical] cycle or proportion? THE COUNT: When a girl is seven years of age, the energy of the circle of the kidneys is abundant, her hair grows, and she gets her second teeth. At twice seven years comes the onset of the natural cycle; the energy flow in the *sinarteria respondens* is now continuous, the energy in the *sinarteria impedimentalis* is abundant, she begins to get her monthly periods and is now capable of bearing children. At three times seven years the active energy of the circle of the kidneys is abundant to the point of spilling over, which causes the wisdom teeth to break through and the long bones to reach their fullest growth. At four times seven years the sinews [i.e., muscles, tendons, and ligaments] as well as the bones have attained their full strength, the growth of the hair is at its most luxuriant, the body is full and round and vigorous. At five times seven years the energy in the *sinarteria splendoris yang* begins to fail; wrinkles appear on the face, and the hair begins to fall out. At six times seven, the energy of the *sinarteria respondens inanis* and the *sinarteria impedimentalis* begins to fail and to diminish, the heavenly cycle is exhausted, and one can no longer walk in earthly ways, so that one's physical form begins to fail and one's capacity to bear or beget children is no more.[8]

Though the count's answer seems relatively straightforward, even allowing for a number of unfamiliar technical terms, the second part of the Yellow Prince's question may still seem puzzling. What he means by "Is this the effect of some natural [numerical] cycle or proportion?" is, essentially, "Is there some inherent property in a particular number of sequence of numbers that puts a stop to one's childbearing ability after one has lived for so many years?" This in turn is connected to the fact that numbers in Chinese culture tend to have qualitative rather than (or in addition to) quantitative significance—which is carried over, for example, in the pidgin expression "number one" for "the best there is" and "number ten" for "the worst." At the very least, things are qualified (rather than quantified) with a number to give them a special emphasis or rhetorical impact, even if the numbers are not thought to have a particular meaning in themselves. We have already encountered the five transformation phases, the six climatic excesses, the seven emotions, and the eight diagnostic criteria. This habit of speech has persisted into modern times so that Mao's antipollution drive, for example, was referred to as "the campaign against the three effluents" (solid, liquid, and gaseous pollution), and here the number three still has more of a

244   qualitative (i.e., "every possible form of pollution") than a quantitative function.

We have tried to show how a medical text can be elucidated, at least in part, by referring to an underlying system of thought—Taoism, in this case—but we are hardly in a position to deny that there are many passages, even entire volumes, in the Chinese medical literature that consist entirely of rootless speculation, deliberate obscurantism, superstition, and out-and-out nonsense. (We will shortly be examining the reason why lapses of this sort became increasingly typical of the literature as a whole as time went on.) And, in any case, we feel that what is superfluous and erroneous in this literature—as well as what is truly worthwhile—can be evaluated only in the context of systematic Chinese medical science and on the basis of a real familiarity with Chinese medical theory.

CONFUCIANISM

If the Chinese predilection for rigorous and acute observation (the pulse diagnostic, for example) was encouraged by the wisdom of the Tao, then it was the Confucianist emphasis on formal speculative thinking that resulted in the emergence of a true medical science. The Confucianists were masters of speculative thought, but since they were primarily concerned with what we would call "interpersonal relations," with ethics and social psychology, they regarded the observation of the natural world as a suitable occupation for a scholar-gentleman's leisure moments at best (and at worst as a complete waste of time).

Clearly, however, the sort of freewheeling speculative thinking that is divorced from all experience (and that has often been characteristic of Chinese thought) is scarcely conducive to the evolution of a rational scientific system. For example, there are three dozen possible sequences or permutations of the five transformation phases, but only three of these are really useful in the context of Chinese medical science—a fact that was determined empirically and could never be ascertained solely by the exercise of pure reason, however ingenious. In general, this is the principal task of science—to select those assertions that are of some practical significance from among the vast number of assertions that are merely "theoretically possible," i.e., that can be formulated with the vocabulary and within the conceptual framework of a particular theory.

Throughout the course of Chinese history (except for a few relatively brief interludes) Taoism has always been identified with those aspects of human experience that could be characterized as elemental, close to nature, chaotic rather than systematic, and frequently also an attitude or state of mind that is asocial, though not necessarily antisocial, but in any case antiformalist. Confucianism was officially enshrined as the ruling philosophy of the empire from 136 B.C. until the year 1905, and though it never completely lost contact with everyday experience in dealing with the sort of ethical or behavioral problems that remained its specialty, the Confucianists preferred to adopt a more strictly rationalist and intellectually formalist approach. The Confucianist bent for speculation, highly refined, not to say effete, served as a kind of counterpoint to the Taoist tradition, a strange blend of mysticism and empiricism that remained vital and more closely attuned to ordinary reality. As a scientific system, Chinese medicine was naturally affected by impulses from both directions but was never decisively won over to one or the other of these rival camps.

Science is never completely divorced from politics, and questions of power play a much greater role than the scientists concerned are generally aware of or prepared to admit. The Confucianists remained effectively in power for the best part of two thousand years, and as far as the Confucianist scholar-bureaucrats were concerned, a physician was nothing more than a more or less skilled craftsman—a repairman, we might say. (This is why the practice of medicine was not a very prestigious calling in imperial China and why a "herb doctor" could never aspire to much more than the equivalent of lower-middle-class status.) It should also not be surprising that very few Confucianists showed much of an interest in medicine, perhaps the most important reason why Chinese medicine developed only very slowly in the millennium that followed the initial compilation of *The Yellow Prince's Classic*. This may also be explained by the not unrelated fact that even the most celebrated doctors tended to be very chary of passing on their skills to more than a handful of students or perhaps no one at all outside their own families.

THE QIN YUERENS: A MEDICAL DYNASTY?

We have already told several anecdotes of the career of Bian Que, the great physician of the second century B.C. and the first physician to have his biography included in the imperial annals—Chapter 105 of the *Shiji* (*Historical Records*), the masterwork of historian Sima Qian (Ssu-ma Chien). In fact, though his fame as a miracle doctor had spread throughout the empire, the annals specifically mention that Bian Que was only the name by which he was known during his lifetime in "the

246 land of Zhao" and that his real name was Qin Yueren. (This is more of a sobriquet than a personal name; it means something like "Emigrant from the Land of Qin," which at that time was a province on the eastern frontier.) Further comparison of the account of his life in the *Shiji* with other surviving sources has led scholars to conclude that there were actually several noted physicians, perhaps an entire family, who bore that name. (One strong piece of evidence for this multiple-Bian Que hypothesis, for example, is that some of his miraculous exploits are reported to have occurred more than a century later than others.) At any rate, the original Bian Que is said to have learned his trade from an old man who took him as his only disciple. "I have formulas for concocting secret remedies," the old man told him. "I am old now, and I will teach them to you as long as you never betray my secrets to anyone else."

However, as we have seen, a great many of the recorded cases of Bian Que emphasize his prowess as a diagnostician. We have already learned how the unfortunate Duke Huan unwittingly brought about his own demise by refusing Bian Que's offer of treatment. On another occasion, Bian Que is said to have arrived at the royal palace in the land of Guo just after the crown prince had lapsed into a coma and had been given up for dead. Suspecting that this might be the case, Bian Que asked to examine the prince's body while it was being prepared for burial. The king of Guo, who was convinced that "my son would still be among the living if you had arrived a little sooner," readily gave his permission. After a brief examination, Bian Que realized that his intuition had been correct. He revived the prince simply by pricking him several times with a needle. After he had been treated with compresses soaked in a decoction of healing herbs, the prince was able to get to his feet and walk away under his own power. Finally Bian Que prescribed a remedy that would fully restore the prince to health by the end of twenty days. Naturally, the story spread abroad among the people of Guo that the foreign miracle doctor was able to raise the dead, but Bian Que modestly demurred: "I cannot bring the dead back to life! The crown prince still had some life left in him; all I could do was find the spark and fan it into a flame, and cause him to awaken and rise from his bed."

According to Sima Qian, "Bian Que became the most famous doctor in all of China. He went to the city of Handan in the land of Zhao, and there he discovered that women were held in particular esteem. Consequently, while in the land of Zhao, he treated the diseases of women." By the same token, he specialized in treating "the complaints of the eyes and ears suffered by old people" while practicing in the gerontophilic city of Luoyang, and in the land of Qin, "where children are held in the highest regard," he naturally became a pediatrician. "Bian Que understood very well that local conditions and the peculiarities of different people must be taken into account." Unfortunately, one human frailty that Bian Que neglected to take into account was the virulent professional jealousy of his colleagues. He was stabbed to death by a hired assassin in the pay of a certain Li Xi, the master of the guild of physicians in the land of Qin.

The name of Bian Que is traditionally associated with two classic medical texts, one of which, referred to in the annals as "a book on the pulse," has not survived. The other is a very important early work called the *Nanjing* (*Classic of Difficult Cases*), which was actually composed around the second century of our own era, or at least four hundred years after the death of the original Bian Que. This at least absolves their ostensible author of any suspicion of having broken his vow to his master never to divulge the secrets of his craft to others, but in fact the anonymous compilers of these early texts must have regarded it as no less serious a breach of the taboos and unwritten laws of their profession to set down this secret medical lore in writing, thus making it available to the merely curious as well as the initiated. (Confucius was among the first to break with tradition in this way by closing the contents of the secret archives of the ruling house he served to his disciples and thus to the world at large.) Perhaps this is another reason why these writers were accustomed to ascribe the authorship of their own works to the celebrated physicians of the past, who were far beyond the reach of censure or reprisal. To be sure, however, it is not impossible that at least some of the contents of the *Nanjing* may have been originally expounded by Bian Que or some member of the Qin Yueren dynasty or even set down in a textbook "on the pulse" by a disciple or some member of his school at least four centuries earlier.

Like *The Yellow Prince's Classic,* the *Nanjing* consists of eighty-one chapters; the first twenty-one are concerned with the pulse diagnosis, the remainder with acupuncture and sinarteriology and the rules of diagnosis in general. The *Nanjing* provides an excellent example of the Confucianist or systematizing trend in Chinese medical literature, insofar as the numerous "difficult" pathological and physiological problems presented in the second section are treated from a strictly theoretical perspective. Chapter Forty-seven, for example, poses this question: "How does it happen that of all the parts of the body only the face is resistant to chills?" It provides this answer: "The head is the chief

248 collecting point for all *yang* [energy]. All the *yin* pathways go only as far as the neck and then turn back down to the breast; only the *yang* pathways lead up to the head. This is the reason why the face has this ability to resist the cold."

ZHANG ZHONGJING (ZHANG JI)

Zhang Zhongjing, still revered in modern times as the greatest of the "sages of medicine," is also the first of the medicine kings who can be confidently identified as the author of an extant medical text, namely the *Shanghan Zabinglun (Treatises on Algor-Induced Disorders)*, the earliest known work on clinical medicine in Chinese. Zhang was born in A.D. 150, passed his scholarly examinations in 168 (which made him eligible for a post in the imperial civil service), was appointed governor of the city of Changsha in 190, and remained there for a number of years. He died in the year 219. He was known for his lofty sense of professional ethics as well as his encyclopedic knowledge of medicine; as a scholar-mandarin, he denounced the low standards of education that prevailed among his medical colleagues and was no less candid in pointing out the shortcomings of his patients as he saw them. Of course, this did not prevent his colleagues' practices from flourishing, though it may well have had an adverse effect on his own.

The *Shanghan Zabinglun* was still required reading for apprentice doctors throughout East Asia during the previous century. It is unique among early medical texts for its methodological, as opposed to theoretical, orientation; the work is actually a compilation of twenty-two separate monographs, which contain some four hundred different practical maxims on the treatment of various illnesses. The term *shanghan* (literally, "harmful colds") that appears in the title may refer to such life-threatening infectious diseases as typhus as well as the more commonplace manifestations of *algor*. Zhang's diagnostic and therapeutic recommendations are expressed in terms of a threefold cycle of *yin* and *yang* derived from *The Yellow Prince's Classic*. The complete sequence consists of a young *yang*, a mighty *yang*, and a "*yang* in eclipse," followed by a young *yin*, a mighty *yin*, and a "yielding *yin*." The *Shanghan* also contains formulas for preparing 113 different herbal remedies, almost all of which are still prescribed today (especially by practitioners of the school of traditional Japanese medicine known as *kampo*, which has also experienced a considerable revival since the beginning of this century). Zhang is also noteworthy as a pioneering advocate of what we would call physiotherapy today, including steam baths, hydrotherapy, and colonic irrigation. ("Find yourself the gall bladder of a boar pig," begins one of Zhang's pharmaceutical recipes. "Mix the gall with some vinegar. Take a section of bamboo about three or four inches long. Insert it halfway into the patient's rectum and pour the mixture into the bamboo.")[9]

Zhang is known to have written a number of other works—treatises on diagnostic technique, gynecology, the pulse, and dentistry—but none of these has come down to us. We owe the survival of the first six of the original ten volumes of the *Shanghan* to the diligence of a physician named Wang Shuhe, who copied them out in about the year 280. Many years later it was discovered that another work attributed to Zhang Zhongjing, picturesquely titled *Particular Rarities from the Golden Shrine*, was identical with the four missing volumes of the *Shanghan*.

HUA TUO

Zhang's contemporary Hua Tuo (c. 141–203) is not associated with any surviving medical text, and he owes his inclusion on the roll of the ancient medicine kings solely to his fame as a practitioner. His name, which sounds somewhat outlandish to Chinese ears, suggests that he was of Central Asian origin, and he seems to have been a strong and highly individual personality, as this anecdote certainly implies:

> A district prefect had been dangerously ill for some time. Hua Tuo was convinced that he could only be cured if he could be induced to fly into a rage for some reason, and accordingly Hua Tuo mulcted him of a handsome fee for the consultation and then simply took himself off, leaving a churlish and insolent letter behind. The prefect was naturally incensed by this high-handed behavior; he sent someone after Hua Tuo to kill him on the road, but Hua Tuo was not to be found. When he learned of this, the prefect flew into a perfect transport of rage, vomited, and recovered straightaway.[10]

Like Zhang Zhongjing, Hua Tuo was also a firm believer in the virtues of hydrotherapy, though in this respect as well his methods were both unorthodox and extreme. On one occasion he is said to have ordered a feverish patient to be put into a bathtub and douched with cold water no less than a hundred times (in spite of the fact that the weather was already very cold). Even though the poor woman was shivering violently, he insisted that the treatment be carried out to the last bucketful. Only then was the patient allowed out of the bathtub—at

250   which point she was bundled up in an especially warm quilt, whereupon
she began to sweat copiously and before long regained her health.

Hua Tuo had also evolved his own system of especially vigorous
calisthenics, the prophylactic and therapeutic benefits of which he
explained in these terms:

> Everyone has the desire to engage in certain activities, but few
> attain mastery. When one is physically active, the energy that one
> takes in with one's food becomes available for use, the bodily fluids
> can circulate without hindrance, and sickness cannot take hold of
> one—just like the hinge on the door, which always turns and never
> rusts. The ancient immortals devised certain exercises—bending
> and stretching, imitating the stance of the climbing bear or the owl
> swiveling its head around, as well as rotating the pelvis and flexing
> all of the other joints—in order to keep old age at bay. I, too, have
> devised a method, which I call the Game of the Five Beasts—
> namely, the tiger, the stag, the bear, the monkey, and the bird. My
> method can not only cure certain illnesses, it can also help one to
> attain greater flexibility in the greater and lesser joints. Anyone
> whose body is still full of stiffness after performing the [conven-
> tional] bending and stretching exercises should perform one of my
> beast exercises as well, since then the sweat will break out all over
> his body and he will immediately feel limber again and completely
> relaxed."[11]

This description of Hua Tuo's system of calisthenics is quoted from a
contemporary historical work, *The Annals of the Three Kingdoms,* which
also contains Hua Tuo's official biography. In spite of the reference to the
"bending and stretching exercises" devised by the ancients, this is the
earliest mention of such a system in Chinese literature, clearly a direct
precursor of the various Taoist gymnastic techniques as well as "tai chi"
(*taiji*) and the related martial arts. It is interesting that a series of similar
exercises are depicted with great accuracy and precision on a group of
illustrated scrolls that was unearthed at an archaeological site in China in
1975; these scrolls are also thought to date from the period of the Three
Kingdoms, which makes them more or less contemporaneous with Hua
Tuo's beast exercises.

Hua Tuo's most remarkable innovation, however, was the discovery
of a potion containing cannabis and other resins and other, unknown
ingredients that could be used as an anesthetic and that thus permitted

him to perform simple surgical operations: "If the illness had settled in the belly or the gut, Hua Tuo would open up these organs and flush them out [with a decoction of various drugs applied to the affected region]."[12] He is also said to have performed a partial splenectomy on several occasions. The incision was stitched up with a medicated suture and healed over within five days; the patients had completely recovered after thirty days. To achieve such results as these, Hua Tuo must also have used an antiseptic of some kind, though here the chronicles do not even give us a hint of what this might have been. (It is curious to note that though Hua Tuo was also an expert practitioner of acu-moxa-therapy and easily the most unorthodox of the classical medicine kings, the analgesic possibilities of the acupuncture needle do not seem to have occurred to him. Today when certain Western practitioners of acuanalgesia try to assert that theirs is one of the "ancient healing arts," such claims must be regarded as having been made in much the same spirit in which the medical writers of classical times were inclined to father their own theories and observations on the Yellow Prince or some other ancient immortal.)

The most famous incident in Hua Tuo's surgical career involved the removal of a poisoned arrowhead from the arm of a great warlord, Duke of Cuan, an episode in which the fortitude of the patient was even more worthy of note than the skill of the surgeon. First Hua Tuo explained that all of the flesh around the wound would have to be excised "down to the bone" to get rid of the poison and that this procedure would obviously be very painful. At this, according to the chronicle,

> The duke cried out, "As long as that's all there is to it!" And he called for wine and drank with his guests. . . . After he had drained two beakers of wine, he lay down on his couch again to resume a game of chess that he was playing with Ma Liang. The duke stretched out his wounded arm, and Hua Tuo took up a sharp knife while his assistant held out a broad basin to catch the blood. "I am about to begin," said Hua Tuo, "but Your Grace should have nothing to fear." "Do what your art requires you to do," the duke replied. "And do you take me for a common sort of rogue, that I might be afraid of pain?"
>
> Thereupon Hua Tuo took his knife and cut down through skin and muscle down to the bone, which was already bluish and discolored. Then he began to scrape off the bone with his knife, which produced a loud grating sound. While everyone else in the

tent turned pale and looked away, the duke called out for meat and wine, carried on his chess game while conversing animatedly, and did not even show the slightest sign of any pain. Finally, after some time, when the blood streaming from the wound had almost filled up the basin, Hua Tuo had removed all the poison, applied a dressing to the wound, and closed up the incision. The duke got up, laughing loudly, and said to his officers, "I can still stretch out my arm as easily as before. There is absolutely no pain. This Master Hua Tuo is truly a divine healer!"[13]

The chronicle goes on to relate that Hua Tuo eventually became the personal physician to the viceroy Cao Cao, the most powerful man in all the Three Kingdoms. However, Hua Tuo began to suffer terribly from homesickness and, offering the pretext that he had a number of pressing family matters to attend to, he deserted his post at court and refused to return. The viceroy found it impossible to persuade him to come back, finally lost patience with him altogether, and, in spite of an attempt by one of the highest court dignitaries to intercede on Hua Tuo's behalf, had him condemned to death. By this point Hua Tuo had realized that the viceroy had been mortally offended by his dereliction of duty and that there was no possibility of a reprieve. "With the hour of his death at hand, Hua Tuo wanted to entrust a medical scroll to the governor of the prison, but he would have nothing to do with it for fear of reprisals. Rather than pressing him any further, Hua Tuo made a fire and burned up all that he had written."[14] Assuming that this story was not simply invented in order to *explain* the fact that Hua Tuo had left nothing behind him in writing, then it seems especially regrettable that this manuscript of his did not survive, since Hua Tuo's medical testament would be likely to contain a great deal that was far outside the mainstream of systematic medical theory and was accordingly not to be found in any of the classical texts.

HUANGFU MI

Hua Tuo was said to have regretted all his life that he owed his fame "entirely to his skill in the healing arts," since though a "miracle doctor" was himself almost revered as a demigod, the guild of physicians as a group still occupied one of the lower rungs of the social ladder. Huangfu Mi could have suffered no such regrets, since he was a respectable Taoist scholar who owes his inclusion in the medical pantheon solely to the fact that he was the author of a volume titled *Zhenjiu Jiayjing* (*Systematic*

Classic of Needles and Moxa), which still has some value as a basic text on
acu-moxa-therapy. Like most works of its kind, the *Zhenjiu* derives its
theoretical perspective from *The Yellow Prince's Classic* and may be
regarded as essentially a compilation of all the authoritative writings on
the subject that had appeared up to that time (late ninth century A.D.).
Huangfu Mi describes 354 different impulse points, gives a great many
detailed technical instructions, and provides a precise symptomology of
the various disorders that can be profitably treated with acu-moxa-
therapy. (Interestingly enough, there is even a supplementary section
devoted to the *foramina* that should *not* be stimulated with needles or
moxa.)

WANG SHUHE

We have already encountered Wang Shuhe (c. 265–317) as the scholar
responsible for the preservation of the first six volumes of the *Shanghan
Zabinglun,* though he is best known as the author of the *Mojing* (*Pulse
Classic*), the first systematic description of the pulse diagnostic and that
presumably represents a distillation of a considerable body of technical
information that had hitherto been transmitted orally from teacher to
student. In this work, Wang Shuhe has also tried to supply a more
thorough explanation of certain basic problems in pathology, much as
Zhang Zhongjing had done in the previous century. It is particularly
striking that the terminology he uses in the *Mojing* has scarcely changed
at all in the intervening sixteen centuries, but the diagnostic techniques
described really have little to do with the rational medical discipline of
pulsiconography as it is practiced today. The conceptual basis of the pulse
diagnostic has clearly undergone a process of considerable refinement
and clarification since the days of Wang Shuhe, and as a result the
Mojing is of no great value as a medical text, though still of interest to the
historian of science.

THE ZHUBING YUANHOULUN

This encyclopedic work, whose title translates as *Notes on the Origins and
Courses of All Diseases,* was prepared by a panel of doctors at the request
of one of the Tang emperors and under the direction of the noted scholar
Chao Yuanfang. The *Zhubing,* consisting of fifty chapters with entries
describing the differential diagnosis and prognosis for as many as 1,720
different disorders, was prepared in a relatively short time for a work of
such impressive dimensions; the first presentation copy was set before the
imperial throne in the year 610. This work was to have an enormous

254   influence on Chinese medicine for many years to come (even down to the present day in certain respects), not only because it was compiled and edited with scrupulous care but also because it was copied and distributed at state expense. This was the first of many such official compilations of current scientific knowledge—state-sponsored encyclopedias, in effect—that have appeared at regular intervals throughout Chinese history. The virtually all-inclusive nature of the *Zhubing* has provided modern scholars with a panoramic view of the state of Chinese science and medicine in this period, as well as a reliable basis for comparison with developing medical sciences in other parts of the world (notably as practiced by the heirs of the Greco-Roman tradition in the Islamic world and the West). The *Zhubing* contains, among many other things, a clearly recognizable description (from the methodological standpoint of Chinese medicine, of course) of smallpox, bubonic plague, measles, and dysentery, as well as the first scientific description of the symptoms and environmental factors associated with beriberi (a vitamin-deficiency disease found primarily in areas where rice is the staple grain crop).

SUN SIMO

Classical Chinese medicine may be said to have reached its zenith in Sun Simo, the last great representative of the esoteric medical tradition. He is said to have lived for a hundred years, from 582 to 682, and the few fragmentary accounts of his life that have come down to us agree that he preferred to live the life of a Taoist hermit-sage in a remote mountain pass than to take up a comfortable post at the recently established academy of medicine. In certain ways, however, Sun Simo was very much in sympathy with the spirit of this newfangled academic medicine, since he devoted his long years of seclusion to the preparation of a vast synthesis of all existing medical knowledge rather than the instruction of a few disciples.

Sun Simo's masterwork, titled the *Qianjin Yaofang* (*Vital Prescriptions Worth a Thousand Gold Pieces*), begins with a discussion of the proper preparation for a career as a physician and of professional ethics, followed by a series of chapters on basic diagnostic and therapeutic principles, the collection and preservation of herbs and medicinal plants, and the preparation and administration of drugs. The remaining twenty-nine chapters are devoted to various medical specialties—something of an innovation for the period—beginning with gynecology (including recommendations for promoting conception), diseases of the eyes and ears, dentistry and mouth disease, and orbisiconography. There is even a section on first aid—emergency treatment of burns and snakebite, fainting spells, and sudden illnesses in general—followed by a more detailed discussion of pharmacotherapy and a section devoted to various aspects of what we would call preventive medicine, including a discussion of macrobiotics and good nutrition, household sanitation, massage, gymnastics, and various techniques for sustaining and replenishing the body's reserves of *qi* (including sexual hygiene and breathing exercises).

Finally, this massive compendium concludes with a discussion of acupuncture and the pulse diagnostic, followed by a kind of theoretical abstract in which Sun Simo incorporates both Taoist mysticism and Confucianist speculative thought and that includes a detailed presentation of transformation phase dynamics and the relatively recently developed doctrine of the influence of climatic and temporal cycles on the origin and course of an illness. To complete the package, a number of Sun Simo's formulas for preparing remedies and other therapeutic recommendations also rely heavily on the Taoist esoteric tradition (magic and alchemy) and on folk medicine. All in all, it seems fair to conclude that Sun Simo had achieved his ambition of distilling all existing medical knowledge, of whatever philosophical persuasion, into a single comprehensive and definitive work. He also anticipated a number of future developments in Chinese medicine—the subdivision of medical science into several different areas of specialization, for one, which was already an accomplished fact at the imperial academy of medicine by the end of Sun Simo's lifetime.

Under the Tang emperors of the seventh and eighth centuries, Chinese culture in general was entering a very eclectic phase, which resulted in a golden age of the arts and letters and, in medicine, a spirit of extremely broadminded tolerance toward any remedy or procedure that was alleged to be of some benefit. The Chinese were also more than usually susceptible to foreign influences and innovations during this period; of the million inhabitants of the Tang emperors' capital, for example, more than a quarter of them were of Central Asian stock (primarily Turkic)—another factor that contributed to the enrichment of Chinese cuisine, artistic motifs and handicrafts, and medicine as well. Sun Simo lists a total of 863 different remedies "worth a thousand gold pieces," which is two hundred more than were in use just 250 years earlier; the newcomers were qualitatively significant as well, since among them, for example, we find the first written description of the medicinal

256   root *Dichroae* (*changshan* in Chinese), which had only recently been introduced from Central Asia and which was among the most effective malaria remedies in the traditional Chinese pharmacopoeia.

SYSTEMIZATION AND DECLINE OF CHINESE MEDICINE

In the heroic age of Chinese medicine, when masters of its esoteric doctrines jealously guarded their knowledge from all but their own disciples, competent physicians were in especially short supply and were naturally much sought after by the princes and great men of the land (as we have already seen in the case of the unfortunate Hua Tuo). During the brief ascendancy of the Sui emperors and once again under the later Tang emperors, an imperial medical office was established in the capital under the auspices of the academy of medicine that we have already mentioned. For the most part, both of these bodies seem to have led a fairly precarious existence and were dissolved and then reconstituted several times over. The medical office was chronically understaffed, and the academy seems to have existed primarily to ensure a steady supply of trained physicians to attend to the emperor and his retinue.

All this was changed under the Sung Dynasty, however, when the practice of all the arts and sciences, including medicine, came to be closely supervised by the imperial bureaucracy. An autonomous body called the Taiyiju ("Great Medical Authority") was established in 1078 and presided over a kind of silver age of Chinese medicine in which a thousand-year-old intellectual and technical tradition was encouraged to reach full maturity under the patronage of the state. The Taiyiju sponsored a medical school that could accommodate three hundred students and the equivalent of a university press in which both classical and more recent works (many of which had previously circulated only in manuscript copies) were carefully edited and reissued in inexpensive printed editions. This unprecedented opportunity for scholarly collaboration and competition seems at first to have had a very stimulating effect on the development of medical science. It is also worth noting that the resident scholars at the academy, like the medical students, were obliged to sit for very rigorous examinations every year.

The Taiyiju also acted as a central clearinghouse for drug formulas and folk remedies from all over China, which were tested and, if proven effective, included in one of the herbals or the official pharmacopoeia that was published by the academy press. This press also occasionally published monographs on a wide variety of specialized subjects—

pharmacology, pathology, pediatrics, obstetrics and gynecology, acu-moxa-therapy, and forensic medicine, to name only the most prominent. Provincial medical offices were established in the provincial capitals, on the model of the Taiyiju, though it is curious to note that in spite of this attempt at centralization and standardization of academic medicine, the medical profession itself remained, as before, completely free of such constraints—which meant that the proportion of competent and thor-oughly trained doctors remained quite small in comparison to the legions of pill-peddlers and traveling mountebanks who shrilly proffered their services in every marketplace.

Another problem with this system, admirable though it was in principle, was that after a century or two it began to succumb to a number of different institutional maladies that would eventually prove fatal to the further development of classical Chinese medical science. Some of the system's real accomplishments—the concentration of China's foremost scholars in a single institution, the closely supervised curriculum and the competitive examinations, the standard editions of canonical medical texts—would eventually contribute to its decline as well, but in retrospect the first sign of trouble seems to have arrived in the twelfth to the fourteenth centuries with the emergence of four distinct schools or factions at the imperial academy, each of which clove to a different segment of the (then still intact) spectrum of therapeutic possibilities to the exclusion of all the others.

This was actually a by-product of the prevailing Neo-Confucianist philosophy of the imperial bureaucracy, which, as we have seen, emphasized purely rational speculation at the expense of empirical observation. The advent of the printed book and the establishment of a centralized repository of "official" medical science in the Taiyiju seems only to have confirmed the ascendancy of a secondary scholarship over research and clinical observation. The literati of the imperial medical office picked up the unfortunate scholarly habit of recycling new books from old, and medicine became a branch of literature and bibliography rather than an applied science.

It is true, however, that there were certain disciplines that tended to be less adversely affected than others by this highly systematic and antiquarian approach. This was particularly true of pharmacology, which had already been established on a firm foundation during the Sung period by a physician from Sichuan named Tang Sheweni, author of the *Zhenglei Bencao* (*Systematic Pharmacology*), the first revised edition of which appeared in 1159 and contained a description of no fewer than

258   1,740 different remedies. During the next century, Zhang Yuansu, still regarded as the most important member of this school, was the first to correlate drug therapy with orbisiconography and to lay down strict standards for the preparation and administration of remedies. His work was carried on by a number of distinguished physicians and pharmacologists, most notably Li Shizhen (1518–93), who devoted almost thirty years to the preparation of the definitive work on Chinese pharmacology, the *Bencao Qangmu* (*Pharmacopoeia in Sections and Subsections*), making a number of collecting trips to various parts of China as well as reviewing and evaluating all the voluminous literature on the subject. Altogether he describes 1,892 different remedies, 374 of them for the first time; the *Bencao Qangmu* also includes a discussion of the basic principles of pharmacology, a section on pathology, and a compendium of the clinical descriptions of a number of diseases, as well as over ten thousand prescriptions illustrating the specific applications of the medicinal plants and other substances described earlier. Some two hundred years later a physician named Zhao Xuemin brought out a greatly expanded edition of this work in which 2,608 different remedies are mentioned, a total that was never to be surpassed in the subsequent literature on pharmacology.

It is perhaps not surprising that the gradual decline of Chinese medical science—characterized as it was by an increasingly pronounced separation between academic and clinical medicine—was also accompanied by a corresponding (and during the last few centuries a dramatic) deterioration in the general health of the Chinese population. For example, even though a technique of immunization against smallpox had been discovered as early as the eleventh century (not vaccination strictly speaking, since it involved the inhalation of pulverized smallpox scabs), no attempt was ever made to eradicate or control the repeated and disastrous onslaughts of this and a great number of other infectious diseases on the masses of the Chinese people. Chinese medicine, as we have learned is most effective when an illness can be immediately detected and treated promptly; the majority of patients, who could not afford a doctor or had to content themselves with the ministrations of a shaman or a charlatan pure and simple, quickly reached the point beyond which medicine could no longer be of any help to them. What is more, as the Russian visitor Tartarinoff was not alone in observing, the medical profession itself had already reached a state of virtually complete demoralization and decadence by the middle of the last century.[15]

The Impact of the West and the Response

VACCINATION was reintroduced into China during the second half of the nineteenth century, along with scientific standards of hygiene and public health. The handful of Western doctors and medical missionaries responsible for these innovations were naturally able to score spectacular successes in the battle against infectious disease, and the superiority of Western over classical Chinese medicine seemed to have been proven beyond all possibility of dispute. In the last years of the empire, the imperial medical office was abolished for the last time, and when in 1914, two years after the proclamation of the republic, a group of practitioners of traditional medicine petitioned to establish their own professional association, they were curtly informed by the new minister of education, "I have decided to forbid the practice of traditional medicine, as well as the traffic in herbal remedies.[16]

The founder of the republic, Dr. Sun Ixian (Sun Yat-sen), had received his medical training in Western-style medical colleges sponsored by the British and Americans in Canton and Hong Kong, and the Nationalist regime officially espoused the cause of the "new medicine," in which the students in the new government-supported medical schools were expected to demonstrate their competence exclusively (though, as we have seen, a parallel attempt to abolish all "indigenous curative practices" was conspicuously unsuccessful). At any rate, since the government was certainly in no position to replace the intransigent herb doctors with trained practitioners of the new medicine, whose services for the most part were available only to the more prosperous inhabitants of the larger cities, the real outcome of this dispute was academic, and for the vast majority of the Chinese people, things continued to go on very much as they had before.

We have already described the series of events—stemming from Mao's decision to enlist all available medical personnel "to serve the

260   people" during the civil war of the 1930s—that ultimately led to a proclamation by the Central Committee of the Chinese Communist Party on November 18, 1958, that henceforth both traditional and modern medicine "should serve side by side." This established the formal equality of the new and the old medicine (in legal and institutional, if not in numerical terms) and has since resulted in the current two-track system of medical education in China, whereby medical students select an area of concentration and devote four of their five years of medical training to the study of Chinese or Western medicine, according to their choice.

At the same time that this directive was issued, doctors in the People's Republic were being encouraged to develop a synthesis of traditional and Western medicine, and it is perhaps only a measure of their success that the most promising hybrid that has resulted from this campaign— acuanalgesia—has become hopelessly confused (in the Western mind, at least) with its Chinese parent, acupuncture. A pamphlet titled *Acupuncture Anesthesia,* published in China in the early 1970s, describes how this upstart child first came into the world: "The throat of a patient in the First People's Hospital in Shanghai was so painfully constricted that he could no longer swallow after he had had his tonsils removed. Personnel of the ear, nose, and throat division inserted an acupuncture needle in the *foramen valles coniunctae* [an impulse point on the *sinarteria intestini crassi* that is on the back of the hand], and the pain immediately stopped. The patient had no difficulty in eating a plate of dumplings shortly afterward. For the medical workers involved, this was a genuine revelation; they began to wonder, since the acupuncture treatment had gotten rid of the pain, if it could also stand in for the anesthetic during the actual tonsillectomy."[17] This supposition, of course, later proved to be correct.

Since most Chinese doctors are familiar with acupuncture, and since anesthetics are expensive and in chronically short supply, this procedure was quickly adopted in other hospitals in Shanghai, and then all over the country. During the Cultural Revolution it became the centerpiece of the internal propaganda campaign for a purely "proletarian science," and an operating theater where major surgery was being performed with the help of acuanalgesia became an obligatory attraction for every delegation of foreign journalists, doctors, or ordinary tourists. It became clear before very long that the greatly inflated claims that were being made on behalf of acuanalgesia were certain to provoke a corresponding backlash of skepticism and disbelief, but there is certainly no good reason to place much credence in more recent reports dismissing "acupuncture anesthesia" as a "propaganda hoax" that has been "discredited and debunked" in China under the current regime.[18] (It is true, however, that acuanalgesia is currently practiced on a much more restricted scale in China. As a member of a medical delegation from the Max Planck Society that went to China in late 1978 at the invitation of the Chinese Academy of Science, I can report that of more than a dozen operations we witnessed, only two or three were carried out with the help of acuanalgesia.)

At the same time, the numerous experiments along the same lines that have been conducted in West Germany and the United States for the past dozen years or so obviously cannot be as easily dismissed as a propaganda hoax. Acuanalgesia has been used as a supplement to more conventional anesthetics in more than a thousand operations—though it is no longer seriously maintained by anyone in the West (or in China) that acuanalgesia can be freely substituted for chemical anesthesia in every case. In cases where the exclusive use of chemical anesthesia might significantly reduce the patient's chances of surviving an operation (e.g., where the patient has a serious cardiac problem), electroacupuncture has come to be used almost routinely in conjunction with a correspondingly diminished dosage of the conventional anesthetic.

BACK TO THE CLASSICS

The twentieth-century revival of traditional medicine in China has not been accomplished without encountering some resistance, nor was it simply a case of "the people lead, the leaders follow," as Mao's propagandists occasionally claimed. In fact, traditional medicine had largely been the preserve of mediocrities and charlatans for a great many years, and there were hardly enough teachers and competent authorities available to reestablish traditional medicine at the level of routine general practice (let alone to bring it up to meet the pedagogical and methodological standards of Western medical science). At the end of the 1940s only a few thousand doctors in China had thoroughly mastered the classical healing arts (a few hundred of these doctors are still active today). A number of working groups of these "veteran doctors" (*laozhongyi*) were formed, and the principal result of their collective labors has been that invaluable series of medical texts that began to appear in the late 1950s, which included a series of textbooks newly compiled for the edification of a new generation of Chinese doctors as well as an annotated standard edition of the classical medical texts.

A survey of the modern literature on Chinese medicine really lies

262   beyond the scope of this volume, but I would at least like to mention one of the first and most distinguished of these works, the *Zhongyixue Gailun* (*General Presentation of Chinese Medicine*), which was prepared by a group of *laozhongyi* at Nanking Academy and published in 1958. I wrote several different reviews of this book (which appeared in various German-language periodicals about a year or so later), since it seemed to me to be a work that had miraculously repaired the ravages of several hundred years and for the first time provided us with a balanced, comprehensive, and authoritative overview of the subject. It seemed no less miraculous that a work like this could be published in the year 1958 without so much as a sidelong glance in the direction of Western medicine (though it may be that I was making a virtue of what had merely been a necessity and that the Nanking veteran doctors had been motivated by honest ignorance of Western science rather than self-restraint).

And as a matter of fact, this quality was perceived as a defect by readers in China who did have some acquaintance with Western science, and in subsequent editions certain concessions have been made to their appetite for modernity. By the early 1970s and the beginning of the Cultural Revolution, the editors' presentation of the principles of Chinese medical theory had come to rely quite heavily on Western concepts and terminology. Over the next few years it became clear that this tendency could only prove self-negating (either politically or epistemologically), and since the late 1970s a certain disillusionment with this approach has become apparent. However, the basic problem remains that the Chinese must find some way of reconciling their intellectual heritage with the exigencies of modern Western science (as far as both methodology and terminology are concerned). And since this is not primarily a scientific but an epistemological and linguistic problem, the Chinese themselves may actually be at a disadvantage when it comes to providing a solution—since, as Whorf was probably the first to recognize, our intimate familiarity with the world view and linguistic backdrop of our own culture may make it all the more difficult for us to gain the necessary distance or perspective required to analyze it in the appropriate methodological and epistemological terms.[19] In any case, it is our good fortune (perhaps one might even call it an unfair advantage) that we may be in a better position to achieve the sort of overview of Chinese medical science that is required—from the complementary vantage point of Western science and Western epistemology (and the territory to be surveyed, of course, has already been set out before us in the *Zhongyixue Gailun*).

In 1959 I embarked on the project of translating this work and quickly discovered that, with the vocabulary at my disposal, I could indeed translate the Chinese words of the text but not the thoughts they expressed, and certainly not the scientific observations they embodied, into a Western language. This left me with three alternatives, namely: (1) to prepare a translation that might be "accurate" and "authentic" by current philological standards but essentially useless as a handbook of practical medicine; (2) to attempt a "free translation" or paraphrase, following the attractive example of a number of well-respected specimens of pseudoscientific chinoiserie, which would undoubtedly appeal to a certain readership as well as the more venturesome practicing physicians; or finally (3), the most difficult and complex of these three alternatives and the only one that I felt justified in choosing, to conduct a thoroughgoing inquiry into the basic epistemological premises of Chinese science and to devise some sort of terminology that would be appropriate to the inductive-synthetic mode of thinking and the functionally oriented assertions that are characteristic of Chinese medical science. This is a task with which I have occupied myself for the past twenty years or so and that I still regard as far from being accomplished.

VIII

THE CURRENT SITUATION

Chinese Medicine and Modern Science

LET us turn once again to Whorf's prophetic warning to the Western scientific community, originally published in 1942: "It needs but half an eye to see that in these latter days that science, the Great Revelator of modern culture, has reached, without having intended to, a frontier. Either it must bury its dead, close its ranks, and go forward into a landscape of increasing strangeness, replete with things shocking to a culture-trammeled understanding, or it must become, in Claude Houghton's expressive phrase, the plagiarist of its own past."[1] Still, however dismal the alternative might be, a nuclear physicist of the present day is unlikely to be greatly cheered by the prospect of following in Whorf's linguistic footsteps and learning Hopi or Shawnee as a way of achieving a fresh, multivalent, and non-culture-bound understanding of the natural world.

Certainly he or she might reasonably object that this project becomes even less feasible if Whorf's prescription is to be applied to the entire scientific community. What scientist, after all, would prefer to contribute a brick to the bottom row of a new Tower of Babel (to use another of Whorf's favorite images) rather than simply to go on gazing out over the parapet of the currently existing one? And doesn't the fact that such an impressive scientific and technological edifice has *not* risen among any of the cultures commended to us by Whorf also seem to suggest that their languages are simply not well suited to the development of a scientific mode of thought?

It is at this point that Chinese medicine might seem to offer a more attractive alternative than simple resignation or frustration—and here we are referring primarily to its cultural and conceptual deep background rather than its more obvious medical possibilities. First, Chinese medicine is a scientific system of rare consistency and completeness, and second, it is formulated in a language that has virtually nothing in common with

268   the Indo-European languages of which Whorf's Tower of Babel is primarily composed. In this sense, Chinese medicine really is a kind of intellectual treasure trove that has been fortuitously preserved thus far and that we are now in an excellent position to plunder. The point of making such an inquiry, with the help of an unfamiliar and unrelated language, is not, however, to acquire new knowledge but rather *to attempt a rational reconstruction of a preexisting body of knowledge that is already available to us in a mature and fully developed form.*

Unfortunately, though, in this case "available" does not mean "instantly accessible," and the difficulties that would have to be surmounted in the course of such an inquiry are numerous enough (and more or less the mirror reflections of those the Chinese have already encountered in reconstructing their own tradition with a rather different purpose in mind). We have already described how we came to decide that a Chinese medical text could only be satisfactorily presented to a Western audience by taking the most arduous and troublesome of three alternative courses—since we felt that only by shedding some light on the epistemological problems involved and by devising an appropriate Western terminology for Chinese medicine could such a text be made truly accessible and its contents not only of cultural and historical interest but of some clinical and practical benefit as well. The history of the exploitation of acupuncture in the West provides an instructive counter-example to the approach we are advocating here, so perhaps a brief review of its history is in order.

After eliciting in the early nineteenth century a flurry of scholarly activity (that was not unconnected with current theories about mesmerism and animal magnetism), acupuncture was briefly in vogue in France as early as 1840. Interest in the subject waned considerably thereafter, and it was not until 1937 that the first professional society for acupuncturists was founded. After the war, a Frenchman, Soulié de Mourant, did a great deal of proselytizing in several European countries and a number of other such societies were founded, whose total membership numbered no more than a few hundred by the late 1950s. James Reston's account of his experiences as a surgical patient in China first appeared in 1971, and as a result of the ensuing publicity barrage, acupuncture was widely discussed in mainstream medical circles for the first time in over a hundred years. So far, however, acupuncture has still not met with complete acceptance in our institutions of higher learning, in spite of the great interest evinced by the students themselves and the widespread use of acuanalgesia (as a modern, technical spin-off of classical acupuncture) in surgical procedures.

This should not be too surprising when we consider that, both clinically and pedagogically, acupuncture has remained within the province of the practicing physician or (in a few European medical schools) the anesthesiologist. But, as we well know by now, therapeutic acupuncture has nothing to do with anesthesia (and in any case makes up only part of the therapeutic stock in trade of classical Chinese medicine), and the practicing physician may not be prepared, either on the basis of his professional training or his subsequent clinical experience, to reconcile the basic principles and scientific expectations of Western medicine with the theoretical capabilities and clinical accomplishments of Chinese medicine. (In the same way, what we may be tempted to think of as simple prejudice by the critics or "opponents" of acupuncture or any other proposed innovation may be nothing more than an understandable reluctance to engage in the sort of mental exertions that is generally unavoidable before one decides to fight one's way out of an otherwise untenable situation by "unproven" radical means.) We should make clear (and here we are not trying to be ironic) that anyone who is quite satisfied with the current state of Western medicine should naturally be exempted from the rigors of such an intellectual ordeal—provided, of course, that he understands that any opinion, particularly a critical opinion, he expresses about the wisdom of selecting a particular itinerary or destination cannot be expected to weigh very heavily with those who have actually embarked on the journey.

THE SCIENTIFIC RECONSTRUCTION OF CHINESE MEDICAL THEORY

It was the philosopher Wolfgang Stegmüller who pointed out that scientists may behave rationally and still remain "narrow-minded dogmatists" at heart.[2] Anyone who insists that Western medicine provides the only conceivable criteria for the rational organization of a certain kind of knowledge is sure to be spared the trouble of coping with alien ideas and outlandish new systems of thought. However, if we *could* use Western scientific means to substantiate our assertion that Chinese medicine is truly a science, then, far from demonstrating the scientific validity of Chinese medicine, this would really be equivalent to admitting that all the technical accomplishments of Chinese medicine could be duplicated by other means, or in other words, that Chinese medicine is

270   merely reduplicative of Western science and thus entirely superfluous. However, as it happens, traditional Chinese medicine has thus far stubbornly and successfully resisted any such attempt at assimilation, which in itself is a strong indication (though, of course, not actually a proof) of the fundamental autonomy of Chinese medical science.

This does not mean, of course, that the rational reconstruction of Chinese medicine would have to be conducted exclusively in Chinese, though we might expect that the impulse to create such a systemization might have originated in China itself—as was indeed the case with the *Zhongyixue Gailun* and its companion volumes. However, a reconstruction of this kind need not aspire to being definitive or comprehensive; it might simply set itself the task of examining the available literature and winnowing out the obvious errors, purely anecdotal material, and stylistic idiosyncrasies, as well as calling our attention to any conceptual gaps or missing sections in the schematic framework. A rational reconstruction of *The Yellow Prince's Classic,* for example, even in Chinese, might well dispense with the dialogue form and the characters of the prince and the Count of Qi (and it is certainly customary for scholars not only to identify these conceptual lacunae in the works of previous authors but also to fill them in, where possible). It may happen that a quite substantial body of work, when subjected to this process of fractional distillation, may yield up only odd fragments of a thought to our theoretical schema—though, of course, the value of these fragments in themselves is entirely independent of the quality of the rest of their creator's work, which may be nothing but the rankest nonsense. (We mention this rather obvious point only because there is a tendency to stigmatize the authors of Chinese medical texts on the basis of their least creditable utterances, just as some writers have attempted to discredit Chinese medicine altogether on the basis of a handful of fatuous quotations and the questionable practices engaged in by certain Chinese doctors. As we pointed out earlier, we would certainly prefer not to have Western medical science similarly "reconstructed" with the help of a few horrifying anecdotes and maliciously selected excerpts from our medical journals.)

In the People's Republic of China today, theoretical consideration of the existing medical literature is largely concerned with the possible practical applications of traditional medicine in the realm of public health. (At any rate, the sort of basic theoretical questions we are concerned with are implicit in the technical vocabulary and in the Chinese language itself and thus manage to escape further theoretical scrutiny for the most part.) Certainly the Chinese deserve nothing but praise for the scrupulous attention that has been paid to scientific questions in the new critical editions of the classical medical texts, and it seems particularly unfortunate that so few libraries and academic institutions outside East Asia took the trouble to get hold of these volumes while they were still available—now that a number of them have gone out of print once again.

One of the problems of discussing this literature in an Indo-European language, of course, is that these basic theoretical questions must be made explicit and we must be able to produce an appropriate equivalent (or at least an explanation) for Chinese medical terms whose meaning can really be made clear only *in the context of a general exposition of the inductive-synthetic mode of thinking.* (Of course, the same thing holds true, *mutatis mutandis,* for the specialized technical vocabulary of any Western discipline with which the reader is presumed to be unfamiliar.) There is no great difficulty involved in concocting a more or less self-explanatory phrase like "impulse point" or "function circle," a neoclassical coinage like "orthopathy" or "contravection," or in appending a word or two of explanation to an unreconstructed Chinese term like *qi* or *xue*. In our experience, the real difficulty is not in substituting an English, German, or Latin word for a Chinese word but in overcoming a fundamental misconception about the nature of Chinese medicine, namely the naïve and complacent belief that medicine is medicine and nothing more— whether it is practiced by an American, a Chinese, or an Australian aborigine. The holders of this belief are also generally (and erroneously) convinced that they already know more or less all there is that medicine, of any kind, has to offer, while losing sight of the fact that what we are actually concerned with here is not just a collection of clinical (empirical) data but an autonomous, fully developed scientific system—and that a merely approximate understanding of its basic tenets will not suffice. (On the contrary, a thorough mastery of the subject is an absolute prerequisite if one is ever to attempt to apply this knowledge in a practical or clinical connection or to engage in further investigations of this kind.)

An example may clarify this last point somewhat: The term *dongmo* (*pulsus mobilis*) may be adequately rendered as "moving pulse" or "mobile pulse," but this term in itself does not actually *reveal* or convey any of the practical or theoretical knowledge that lies behind it. (In the same way, we would not be prepared to concede that someone had "learned to drive" simply because he had grasped the principle that one is expected to turn a wheel and activate certain levers with his hands and

272   feet.) Practical training, *clinical* preparation, and the ability to apply the principles of Chinese medical theory can begin only when one has made all the essential connections and has extrapolated all the relevant points of knowledge into a coherent rational framework. Aimless experimentation and dilettantism can only lead, at best, to the acquisition of certain purely technical skills (acupuncture, for example, as it is practiced in the West) or to out-and-out fakery and charlatanism.

Suffice it to say, then, that the rational reconstruction of Chinese medicine involves more than just translation, or the substitution of one set of terms for another, since individual theoretical concepts have no meaning in and of themselves but can be defined (and understood) only in terms of all the other elements that make up the technical vocabulary of Chinese medicine. This confronts the student with something of a paradox—rather like trying to unravel a ball of string that appears to have no loose ends. That such an all-or-nothing approach can be successful has, of course, been abundantly demonstrated by the Chinese themselves, since the transition from an inductive-synthetic scientific background to a causal-analytic one is surely no less arduous than the reverse.

There also seems to be an unmistakable if not clearly articulated preference that is beginning to manifest itself in the West today for the inductive-synthetic mode of thought. Certainly the ability to "display" information in "graphic" (i.e., pictorial) or symbolic terms is regarded as a great aid to clarity in cases where a purely verbal description might be impractical or cumbersome. The saying "A picture is worth ten thousand words" (sometimes represented as a Chinese proverb) is increasingly applicable to many of the sciences today, and certainly this is as true in the field of medicine as in any other. Perhaps this implies a mode of perception that simply cannot be expressed in words—though medical historian Gerhard Pfohl has derisively referred to this propensity to be "pictorial at any price" as "the illiteracy of the modern age."[3] If so, then perhaps only a further infusion of inductive-synthetic Chinese thought can help ward off the doom of speechlessness that awaits us.

A number of Western observers, not in themselves particularly well disposed toward Chinese thought, seem to be pleased to report that the Chinese in recent years have been increasingly turning back toward Western causal-analytical thinking and away from their own intellectual heritage. At the moment this is quite true, and it may result, as it has done in the past, in another period of neglect and disparagement of Chinese medicine, which, in our view, would not only be ill-advised and presumptuous but also potentially disastrous. Devotees of Western medicine may at least find momentary distraction in contemplating the problems currently faced by the Chinese medical and scientific establishments, which are precisely antithetical to and certainly no less pressing than our own. Since the mid-nineteenth century, the Chinese have been in the throes of a protracted existential crisis, which followed the abrupt dissolution of the Neo-Confucian system of science and philosophy. (It is worth noting that, given sufficient time, the installation of an established mode of scientific thought eventually gave rise to an intellectual system of unprecedented complexity and rigidity.) For the Chinese, however, the confrontation with Western science and technology has not been merely an abstract philosophical question—involving the mechanical substitution of a "causal-analytic mode" for an "inductive-synthetic mode"—but a question of the survival of a culture. The fact that this conflict is also perceived by many as primarily a question of global power politics need not really concern us here, nor the fact that even a great many Chinese seem to have forgotten that part of what is at stake, at least, is the survival of a mature indigenous science that makes up an important part of that culture. In the West, after all, a similarly nonchalant attitude toward our own indigenous science and technology has been in evidence since the days of Rousseau and has become particularly pronounced in the last decade or two, as represented by the environmentalists and Whole Earth evangelists who are not merely complaining, let us say, of the one-sidedness and the inherent limitations of the causal-analytical outlook but who are also inveighing against Western science and technology with the indiscriminate ardor of the prophets of old.

We have already had occasion to observe in connection with the history of Chinese medicine that true science can flourish only if there is an appropriate balance between empirical observation and speculative thought, by means of which the empirical data so acquired can be constructed into a system. Pure empiricism in the absence of such an organizing principle is merely prescientific thought, and abstract speculation divorced from the precise observation of reality results in a kind of sterile scholasticism (still vigorous enough to perpetuate itself, however, from one generation of scholars to the next).

There can be no doubt that this was the fate of the natural sciences in China between the fourteenth and the nineteenth centuries, but we in the West would be much less freely disposed to admit that a similar outbreak of scholasticism—a form of desiccated hyperintellectualism of unprece-

274 dented virulence—has taken hold among us since the Second World War. The student's imagination and intellectual curiosity is sated quickly enough with triple-distilled fourthhand knowledge that neither his professor nor his professor's professor has actually acquired from his own personal experience or verified with his own eyes. The product is obtained instead from more or less anonymous sources, periodically repackaged and relabeled, thriftily recycled and enriched with freshly synthesized terminology, and of course constantly refined to an ever-higher level of abstraction. Whether this new brand of scholasticism is to be regarded as a deadly scourge or simply another instance of consumer fraud, it seems likely that Western science—and an entire culture that has become more and more dogmatically and insistently identified with it—may be carried off by it much more rapidly than was its Chinese counterpart.

History seldom repeats itself, and this holds true for the history of science as well. But if it is also true that Western medical science is nowadays useful only for the treatment of rare diseases, as Arthur Jores maintains,[4] then surely is it no less divorced from everyday reality, from the real needs of its patients, than Chinese medical science in its most decadent phase? The fact that this process of alienation has been accomplished in the West in a highly disciplined, rational manner, even while subject to the strictest public scrutiny, will not be acceptable as an excuse very much longer.

In many ways, Chinese medicine does appear to be more considerate of its patients' welfare, as in the case of the cumulative side effects of drug therapy, which can be immediately detected as functional aberrations and corrected in the normal course of therapy—whereas in Western medical practice they may not be diagnosed until they have already given rise to a serious organic disorder. Chinese medicine holds itself to a stricter standard of accountability, and even the sages of ancient times were extremely candid in acknowledging the limitations of their art. This means that Chinese medicine is to become—as Arthur Jores has no less candidly acknowledged on behalf of Western medicine—the cause of chronic human misery, and the concept of "iatrogenic illness" (as distinct from out-and-out malpractice) does not exist in Chinese medicine.

The fact that the technique of acuanesthesia that has been developed in West Germany is far less harmful to the patient than the standard chemical anesthetics is no longer seriously disputed, even by those doctors who remain absolutely unconvinced of the benefits of acupuncture therapy. (They may still raise the objection that acuanesthesia is not invariably painless and that we still do not really understand how it works; but of course when we are dealing with prospective patients for whom any kind of chemical anesthetic would be contraindicated, then these objections need not weigh very heavily.) At the same time, the potential public-health and economic advantages, to say nothing of the medical benefits, of traditional Chinese medicine became sufficiently evident to persuade the World Health Organization, an agency of the United Nations, to organize a conference on acupuncture, moxibustion, and acuanalgesia in June 1979 in Beijing (Peking). The delegates drew up a list of over a hundred different disorders that have been successfully treated with acupuncture—though the organizers of the conference were obliged to point out that this list had been compiled on the basis of doctors' testimony rather than independent clinical testing. The WHO endorsement of Chinese medicine may thus be regarded as faint praise (which may have something to do with the fact that not nearly enough clinical investigation of these therapeutic claims has been carried out since then) but cannot be dismissed out of hand—unless one is disposed to believe that an organization like the WHO, often enough the target of criticism and controversy in the past, would go out of its way to issue even a qualified endorsement of herbal magic and sorcery, or, to use more current terminology, "nonspecific contact therapy" and autosuggestion.

THE CHINESE TREASURE TROVE

It was Mao Zedong who first referred to the "vast treasure trove" of Chinese medicine, and in recent years, as never before, like the treasures of the Vatican and the Tower of London, the treasures of Chinese medicine have been readily available for public inspection. A great many Western doctors have taken advantage of this touristic opportunity, but since the duration of their stay rarely exceeds three weeks, the treasures themselves may prove disappointing, displayed as they are in a seemingly heterogeneous jumble in which the trained Western eye can discern no central pattern of organization. A Western doctor in China, however perceptive and adaptable he might be, is still going to perceive human beings as organisms with nerves and blood vessels, tumors and inflamed appendixes—and if he seriously wants to learn to see people as individuals with function circles and arterial pathways through which energy flows according to the periodic cycle of the five transformation

276   phases, then he need no longer go to China to learn to do so in the first place.

One thing that is still apparent to every foreign visitor to the People's Republic of China, irrespective of his attitude toward Chinese medicine (if any), is the good general health of the population—which may still come as something of a surprise to those of us who were first introduced to the Chinese people, through travelers' and missionaries' accounts of some years ago, as plague-ridden and half-starved, victimized by quacks and sorcerers. Certainly the introduction of Western notions of hygiene and public health has had something to do with this remarkable transformation, but bear in mind that Western medicine also enjoyed the full confidence and patronage of the previous regime, but without any very encouraging results. It was only when the resources of traditional Chinese medicine were fully mobilized, as described by Dr. George Hatem, that the medical breakthrough that the Nationalists had vainly hoped for could finally occur.

In more recent years it has become increasingly clear that Western medicine is incapable of providing effective medical care for millions of sick and dying people in the Third World. The indiscriminate use of antibiotics has finally blunted the edge of this powerful weapon against infectious disease; penicillin may currently be doing more to encourage the propagation of drug-resistant bacterial strains than to prevent infection. Doctors and public-health officials in many countries are baffled by the reappearance of malaria, and even the bubonic plague, in areas where these scourges had long been thought to be extinct. In short, Western medicine no longer seems to be capable of delivering on the promises that have been made in its behalf.

The most important implication of the WHO's qualified endorsement of acupuncture is that sick people might be helped by means other than those that have been designated by academic Western medicine. Purists might conceivably object that the list of illnesses that may be treatable by acupuncture therapy was prepared entirely in accordance with the criteria of Western medicine and merely furnishes another example of how difficult it is even for well-informed professionals, favorably disposed toward acupuncture, to make much headway in the alien terrain of Chinese medical science. (Realistically, we must also acknowledge that a comparable list of disorders that had been drawn up according to the criteria of *Chinese* medicine would be perused by the international medical community with blank incomprehension. Systematic Chinese medical science still has many more worlds to conquer.)

The Chinese system of preventive medical care, based on the ubiquitous barefoot doctor, may also provide a model for the delivery of primary health care (though not necessarily in the form of traditional Chinese medicine, of course) throughout the Third World. In the West, in light of several million successful acupuncture sessions, Chinese medicine can be regarded as fairly well established, if not necessarily in its purest form, and it does not take any great gift of prophecy to foresee that it will go on to play a much more important role in the years to come all over the world. There is really no great harm in the fact that practical advances in the field are progressing at so rapid a clip that scientific research will probably continue to lag behind for some time to come (or even allow itself to be carried along for some considerable distance without pulling in briskly on the reins immediately).

And if mainstream medical science is willing to become involved, then it must be prepared to shed all of the prejudices associated with causal-analytical thought, and especially to steel itself against the temptations of intellectual arrogance, in order to follow the trail blazed by Whorf into "a landscape of increasing strangeness, replete with things shocking to a culture-trammeled understanding." No matter how extensive one's knowledge of Western medicine, this still does not qualify one to pronounce on the validity of Chinese medicine, and any assertion of this kind that is based entirely on Western scientific criteria must accordingly be regarded as *disinformation*—i.e., "information" that is neither demonstrably true nor untrue but is presumed to be misleading and unreliable by its very nature. (The same strictures must be held to apply to the collector of intellectual chinoiserie, the seeker after scientific curiosa, who is willing to engage in a flirtation with an exotic scientific creed without ever straying very far away from the formidable chaperon of his own cultural preconceptions. A number of these connoisseurs have taken part in cultural exchange programs with the People's Republic and have returned quite happy to have seen the sights and with all their original prejudices still intact.)

At this point we would like to express the possibly naïve hope that we might be able to shake ourselves free from the grip of cultural prejudice without immediately rebounding to the other extreme and embracing the belief that Chinese medicine is quite simply the "alternative" that is going to free us all from the overmechanized, dehumanized, and megalomaniacal excesses of Western medicine. Actually, to take such a position would be to do less than justice to the genuine capabilities and accomplishments of Chinese medicine. Alternatively, to reject the valid

278   scientific core of Western medical science simply to rid ourselves of the scholastic and mechanistic accretions so frequently and justifiably complained of would obviously represent a great step backward for our own civilization. Our goal is not to exchange our original set of preconceptions for another that is no less one-sided and inflexible, but what we hope to establish is a new kind of medicine that can freely accept the observations and accumulated knowledge of both cultures. For this to occur we must always be particularly mindful of the welfare of those that all medicine is intended to benefit, and we must remain open and receptive to the legitimate claims of any mature medical science.

Afterword
Testing the Safety and
Effectiveness of Drugs: An
Inductive-Synthetic Approach

THE traditional Chinese pharmacopoeia begins to seem like an ever more valuable resource as the safety and effectiveness of Western-style drug therapy come increasingly into question. At present, the consensus seems to be that four fifths of our prescription and over-the-counter remedies simply cost too much and that (a) certain remedies are utterly ineffective whereas (b) others do not have the effects that are claimed for them by their manufacturers or (c) have deleterious side effects that are more pronounced than their primary therapeutic effects so that treatment can be continued for only a relatively short time.

This far from satisfactory situation has been variously blamed on the rapacity of the drug companies, the apathy and inertia of the governmental bodies responsible for regulating such matters, and the indifference and complacency of the medical community itself. It seems that the real cause of this pharmacosocial chaos can be identified with the failure of academic Western medicine (on which these other putative villains, including the practicing physician, all rely as the ultimate scientific authority) to provide reasonable and practical standards for the testing of new drugs before they are allowed onto the market. All the other problems we have alluded to (and thus perhaps a major portion of the current public discontent with the cost and quality of available medical care in the industrialized nations) can be seen to flow from this common source—which for purposes of our discussion may be defined as a somewhat irrational conception of the ways in which drugs affect the human body.

The idea that the effects of a newly synthesized drug should be tested

280 systematically and scientifically was first enunciated at about the beginning of the nineteenth century, when pharmacology itself was first established as an independent scientific discipline (and about the same time as the birth of the modern chemical industry). Not very much was heard of this idea outside of professional and specialist circles, however, until the middle of the twentieth century, when the proponents of the causal-analytic school of chemotherapy made a major effort to have certain therapeutic techniques regarded by them as unscientific legally barred from the realm of medicine. Since then, a number of countries have revised their statutes governing the scientific testing of drugs (which meant that, depending on the relative political power of the parties to this dispute in the country involved, the medical and political status quo was frequently endorsed as being legally and socially desirable as well).

In general, if a drug is defined as a substance that is administered to eliminate, control, or moderate the effects of a pathological disorder, then our principal criteria for measuring the effectiveness of a given drug should simply be whether or not the intended or predicted effects of this drug are routinely and reliably observed, and whether or not there are any significant side effects (and what the extent and intensity of any side effects that are present might be). The testing procedures adopted in accordance with these criteria should be sufficiently precise and unambiguous to detect any significant deviations or irregularities in the first case and sufficiently comprehensive to collect all the relevant data in the second. None of the testing procedures that have thus far been developed under the aegis of causal-analytic medicine has been able to satisfy these basic requirements, and unfortunately those that are currently in use cannot be said even to come close.

THEORETICAL BACKGROUND
The reason for this, we believe, may be described as theoretical rather than technical or practical and thus may be revealed by examining certain underlying intellectual assumptions that are common to all of these procedures—as well as a number of curious intellectual aberrations and irrational dogmas that have grown up in association with them.

We have already observed that the causal-analytic method is primarily concerned with providing a description of a sequence of events that have already taken place and can make scientifically authoritative statements only about phenomena that can be measured—that have a material form available for scientific inspection. In the present context, then, determin-

ing the effects of a given drug means establishing a strict pharmacodynamic correlation between a precisely defined substance and a precisely
defined experimental substrate, namely a group of human subjects (a
particular kind of tissue in a group of living human organisms). As long
as we remain exclusively concerned with this very precisely defined
relationship between a given substance and a measurable somatic
alteration, in effect, then we have had the technical means at our disposal
to perform such a test, in the most stringent and scientifically exacting
fashion, since about the turn of the century. The difficulty here is that, as
we know, the phrase "somatic alteration" implies an entire sequence of
previous *functional* alterations or impulses radiating outward from a
single source. Long before the substance in question has had a chance to
effect a measurable somatic alteration of this kind (either by virtue of a
heightened experimental dosage or prolonged administration of the
drug), it will have already produced a variety of functional alterations in
the test subject's physical and mental activities, including his overall
energy level, routine bodily functions, attitude and psychic state, etc. All
of this, like everything else that may be described as dynamic, functional,
and vital, does not really come within the sphere of competence of a
science that is based on causal analysis.

On the other hand, the practical physician is constantly made aware of
the normal and abnormal fluctuations in his patients' energy levels,
psychic states, and general functional activity. He may first become
aware of an illness as a disruption of the patient's subjective sense of
well-being, perhaps accompanied by changes in his thoughts and feelings
and in the accustomed pattern of his activities, which (as doctor and
patient both know from experience) may lead to more serious somatic
complications later on. The doctor also knows that these functional
deviations from the norm may be alleviated or corrected by means of
certain drugs, but this is something he has discovered on a strictly
empirical basis, in the same way that medical lore of this kind has been
collected and put into practice for thousands of years. As we mentioned
a little earlier, such knowledge can at best be regarded as prescientific; it
may serve as a kind of prelude to (but never as a substitute for) a strict
scientific understanding. Thus there has come to prevail in many medical
practices and hospital wards an uneasy coexistence between a strictly
rational scientific method and a brand of empiricism that is far less strict
and merely reasonable. In the highly specialized world of modern
medicine, the effects of newly developed drugs are tested by clinicians
and pharmacologists who may not be aware of this curious imbalance

282   between an exact science (which operates with a high degree of precision within a very restricted area and is thus optimally effected within that area) and prescientific empiricism, as it still lingers on in the vast, untamed hinterland of practical medicine—or perhaps if they are aware of this discrepancy, they have simply chosen to ignore it.

TECHNICAL CRITERIA FOR A SCIENTIFIC TESTING PROCEDURE

Thus, unfortunately, the procedures currently used in testing the effectiveness of drugs are not generally subject to a salutary empirical corrective of this kind. But even if the immediate and intangible (functional, psychological, perceptual) effects of the drug are largely overlooked, at least in most clinical testing procedures there is an attempt to identify (and thus to manipulate crudely or simply "factor out") the more obvious psychological effects of the experiment in the interests of scientific objectivity.

Most readers are probably familiar with "blind" or "double blind" clinical tests, in which test subjects are divided into two groups, one of which will receive the drug that is being tested, the other a placebo (a capsule filled with milk sugar or some other innocuous substance). The patients are naturally unaware of the substitution, the purpose of which is to enable an obviously troublesome variable—the patient's expectations that the drug will help him to get better—to be factored out of the experimenter's equation. In a double-blind test, the doctors or nurses who administer the drugs are also unaware that certain subjects are being given a placebo (though, of course, they may well suspect that an experiment of this kind is taking place).

We believe that it is simplistic to assume that by figuratively blindfolding both patient and doctor, the potentially disruptive intangible effects of administering the drug—"disruptive" in the sense that they lie outside the extremely narrow compass of the experiment—can safely be ignored. The experimental design is further disfigured by the crude behavioristic assumption that only two of the patient's emotions or nonphysical sensations need be taken into account—namely, hope (that the medicine will help him get better) and fear (that not taking the medicine would make him feel worse). That any of the patient's other thoughts or impressions might have some bearing on the way he feels, might expedite or impede his eventual recovery, never seems to have occurred to the designers of these experiments. The effects of the hospital environment, the bizarre social relations that prevail in such places, the proximity of so much expensive and intimidating equipment (and the fact that different people react to such things in strikingly different ways)—all of these are deemed equally unworthy of consideration. (Finally, before we abandon the subject of double-blind clinical testing, we believe there is one aspect of this procedure that is truly unconscionable rather than merely regrettable. By what conceivable standard of morality could it be permissible for a doctor to offer a patient a worthless sugar pill—or worse, to administer an untried experimental drug—without his knowledge or consent, that could conceivably increase his suffering or even shorten his life?)

At this point we would like to expand on our earlier list of criteria for a scientific testing procedure by positing the additional requirements that the test results should be *positive* (which we will define shortly) and that the test procedures themselves, as befits any legitimate scientific experiment, should be both reproducible and verifiable. By *positive* we simply mean that the test should yield empirical data that will tell us how the drug in question will actually work—that the test conditions will closely approximate the conditions under which the drug might be administered in practice. This may seem like a truism, almost a tautology, but it is in fact a principle that is widely ignored by pharmacologists who attempt to predict the effects a drug will have on human beings on the basis of data obtained exclusively from experiments with animals. Here, as before, the problem is that studies involving mice or guinea pigs or even baboons really tell us nothing about the emotional, perceptual, or the plethora of other *functional* effects that a drug might have on human subjects. It may be of some interest to know that a given dosage of a given drug induces belching or symptoms of euphoria in mice, but in most cases when data of this kind are extrapolated to predict the same drug's effects on humans, the results of these computations cannot be regarded as positive data but merely as an experimental hypothesis (which may or may not be borne out by more appropriate test procedures).

We have already stipulated that the test procedure should be precise and unambiguous in its determination of the effects of the drug in question. This presupposes that the test results should be expressed in terms of a commonly accepted and clearly defined normative convention. This in turn brings us back to a familiar problem: Western medicine cannot really provide us with a sufficiently unambiguous and coherent set of criteria that will enable us to describe a drug's immediate *functional*

284   effects with the necessary precision. (We should point out that all assertions concerning functional activity in Western medicine—in the realm of physiology, for example—are either strictly empirical or, where they are based on precise quantitative measurements, extrapolated from an observable past state to a strictly hypothetical "present.")

Our requirement that the test procedure be comprehensive in scope, though straightforward enough in principle, may also be the most problematical. In reality, *all* the effects that a single drug can produce in an individual may not be measurable or even distinguishable. The effects of a particular substance will vary according to the nature of the substrate with which it comes in contact—which is why experiments with animals or purely analytical experiments carried out *in vitro* are inadmissible for our present purposes. Purely empirical data, however copious, concerning the effects of a drug on an individual subject, or a statistically significant group of subjects, also cannot be regarded as sufficiently comprehensive, since (1) these data are necessarily restricted in their purview to the observer's sensory impressions of a limited series of events and (2) certain key events that are essential to the continuance of our vital processes occur so rarely (opportunities for observing them are severely limited in space or time) that they are unlikely to turn up merely by chance in a straightforward statistical sampling of this kind. To arrive at a conclusion that is sufficiently comprehensive for our purposes, in practical if not in absolute terms, it will be necessary to make conscientious and systematic use of the resources of a particular methodology, rather than leaving such matters more or less to chance.

For example, to determine whether a patient has an elevated white blood cell count, it is simply not enough for us to have a microscope at the ready if we have no idea how to take a blood sample or how to evaluate the relative proportions of red and white corpuscles in the blood—which is part of the methodology that has been developed by causal-analytic medicine for this precise purpose. This point seems all the more relevant if we are interested in determining which individual functions are affected by a given drug, and in what way. To begin with, we will certainly need to have access to a list of all the significant functions, and of course we will also have to be familiar with the technical means by which these predicted functional deviations can be reliably ascertained and described (and we will also want these observations to be readily reproducible). Here again, we know of no other scientific system that provides such a rigorous, subtly differentiated, and practicable means of accomplishing these tasks as Chinese medicine.

A NEW FORM OF TEST PROCEDURE

This would have to fulfill all of our theoretical criteria: It would provide a positive, precise and unambiguous, and comprehensive description of the effects of any substance (or procedure) that was intended to be used for therapeutic purposes. A therapeutic procedure might include some sort of physiotherapy, hydrotherapy, or massage, for example, and the full range of medicinal substances that might be tested extend all the way from homeopathic remedies (which have virtually no "active ingredients" at all, in the conventional sense of the term) through the more traditional phytotherapeutic (herbal) remedies, including herbal extracts and mixed preparations of remarkable complexity and every conceivable provenance, to the simple or complex substances that are employed in chemotherapy and that we customarily think of as "drugs."

The test consists of two or possibly three different stages and may be administered to a large group of subjects, dispersed over a wide geographical area, whose reactions may be monitored over an indefinite period of time. (It is essential, however, that remedies intended for human consumption should be tested exclusively on human subjects.) Earlier model test procedures tended to shy away from running tests on human subjects—and with good reason, since the object of these procedures was to induce actual somatic alterations in the subject. (We might liken this to a hypothetical experiment designed to test the listener's physiological responses to the violin—in which instead of letting loose with a melancholy adagio or a stirring apoggiatura passage, the performer is instructed to beat the subject over the head with his instrument until he has elicited a discernible somatic alteration.) At any rate, any substance can produce a whole panoply of detectable functional effects long before enough has accumulated in the tissue to produce a somatic alteration, and, moreover, these functional effects are completely reversible. (Naturally, the experimenters would begin by administering a dose of the test substance that is several orders of magnitude less than would be required to produce a somatic effect of any kind.)

A Functional Profile of the Test Subject

Since there is no way of judging beforehand how an individual subject might react to a particular substance (and what this reaction implies in terms of the pharmacodynamic criteria of the test procedure), a complete functional profile of every test subject would have to be assembled during the first stage of the test. (This has nothing to do with illness as such, of course, nor does it imply the existence of any functional

286   disorder.) What is being tested for basically comprises everything that might otherwise be categorized by such versatile pseudoscientific catchphrases as "placebo effect," "spontaneous remission," "idiopathic drug reaction," or "autosuggestion." Such a profile can be made complete enough (by using the diagnostic techniques of Chinese medicine) that any instability or transitional "borderline state" that exists in any of the function circles can be detected long before a corresponding physical change of state would have been apparent. This would enable the experimenter to decide, e.g., that a particular test substance should not be administered to a given subject, since this would be likely to cause a disruption of a particularly unstable functional equilibrium, which in turn might cause the subject unnecessary pain or distress. The timely awareness of what we have called a functional borderline state might also enable the experimenter to determine in advance that a somatic alteration in a given subject that would otherwise be misinterpreted as a "positive test result" would have taken place in any case—even if the test substance had not been administered, or alternatively that a false negative result would have been obtained in either case.

The Functiotropic Test

The purpose of this second stage of the test procedure is to assign a qualitative value to the functional effects of the test substance, based on the direction in which orthopathy is "pushed" or "deflected" by repeated administrations of the test substance to a group of healthy subjects over a prolonged period of time. (It is also advisable for the subjects to be volunteers; people who are in pain or who are anxious about their health cannot be said to have "volunteered" to take part in such a test, and accurate recording of all the observations that are required actually involves a considerable expenditure of time and a certain amount of endurance as well. If the long-term effects of a substance are being tested, it might be necessary to keep an individual subject under observation for a period of months, if not years.)

    The observers will begin by taking note of everything in the subject's behavior and demeanor that we have come to designate as the results of "functional activity," including the subject's emotional and psychic state. Remember that the functional effects of any substance or therapeutic procedure are also its primary effects on the individual, which can neither be avoided nor suppressed, and by the time an observer has detected some somatic alteration in the subject, this means that a wide variety of functional factors have already been at work for some time.

The description of these effects must necessarily begin just as soon as the test substance is administered, and very often a final determination of these initial effects can also be regarded as the end result of the entire test procedure—whenever, e.g., a functional disorder that is present at a certain dosage level gives way to potentially deleterious (for which read "toxic") side effects when the dosage is increased.

At least two thirds of the illnesses treated by contemporary medical science may be regarded as functional disorders (in addition to a number of others that are classified as "polyfactorial"). Given that Chinese medicine has already assembled the methodological resources, yet only part of the empirical data that are necessary to diagnose successfully and treat such disorders, would it not seem advisable to supplement the sketchy descriptions of many of the existing Chinese remedies in the current literature by subjecting these (and other traditional remedies, including those of the Galenic pharmacopoeia in the Western tradition) to a rigorous and systematic series of functiotropic tests, as described above?

The Somatotropic Test

The third stage of our testing sequence, as its name implies, is equivalent to the existing test procedures, except that as it would be performed only *after* the experimenter had fully evaluated the results of the previous tests (both of which may be of particular assistance in predicting the occurrence of potentially hazardous side effects). Thus both experimenter and subject will be embarking on this final stage of the test procedure with a great deal more information than they would have had otherwise; we recommend that the subject be briefed on the results of each of the preceding test stages, and also that he be informed in advance of the experimenter's expectations of what the next test stage is likely to reveal in light of previous results.

Some clinical testing will probably be necessary at this stage, particularly if the remedy in question is intended for the treatment of an advanced disorder with pronounced somatic symptoms. Problems involving the side effects of newly developed drugs obviously cannot be avoided altogether, but even here the experimenter will be in a better position to monitor (and predict) the functional effects of the initial dose of the test remedy and thus gradually build up to an effective dosage. It may also be necessary for the test remedy to be buffered (or perhaps fortified) by the addition of some other substance; here a knowledge of the old-fashioned pharmacopoeia and of modern analytical chemistry

288   might not be amiss. Once again, it may be advisable to keep an individual subject under observation (at intervals) for months or even years, a fact that should obviously be explained to the prospective volunteer at the outset.

THE STANDARDIZATION OF REMEDIES

One implication of this new pharmaceutical testing procedure is that remedies (particularly herbal or phytotherapeutic remedies) can now be standardized—i.e., both scientifically classified and therapeutically dispensed—on the basis of their clinical effects rather than their chemical constituents. If this seems like a point that is of strictly academic interest, perhaps a word of explanation is in order. Modern pharmacology has seen fit to standardize all officially recognized remedies according to their active ingredients. (This question does not really arise for the synthesized substances that are used in chemotherapy, which are formally described in terms of the chemical equations that represent the steps involved in their manufacture, including the relative proportions of the various chemical ingredients.) Attempts have been under way since the middle of the nineteenth century to analyze and similarly standardize the effective ingredients of the herbal and other natural remedies in the traditional pharmacopoeia. Consequently in many countries, for example, the drug atropine has an official place in the pharmacopoeia, but the deadly nightshade plant from which it is derived is no longer recognized as a therapeutically effective remedy. A great many practitioners are dissatisfied with this state of affairs, since they believe that the natural remedies often have a broader spectrum of effectiveness than their ostensible "active ingredients" in isolation. Thus far, however, in the absence of any effective pharmaceutical testing procedure, this debate has merely been smoldering inconclusively for some time.

Now we are at last in a position to ascertain the precise clinical effects of even the most complex therapeutic mixture, a fact that should be of commanding interest to both doctors and patients—patients may not be overly concerned with the provenance or chemical composition of whatever medication they happen to be taking, but they generally are quite seriously concerned with the question of its safety and reliability and the relative permanency of its effects. This is precisely the sort of information that is conveyed by the functiotropic testing procedure we have just described. And as soon as there are enough doctors available who are thoroughly familiar with the diagnostic procedures of Chinese medicine, it will finally be practicable (and remarkably inexpensive, by the way) to reclassify and to standardize the majority of these remedies in accordance with their clinical effects rather than their chemical content. (The current system is further complicated by the fact that herbal remedies may vary in strength and effectiveness according to the time of year at which they were gathered, their place of origin, local and seasonal climatic variations, and so on—in much the same way that grapes of the same variety growing in different vineyards in different localities may produce wine that varies remarkably in quality.) And when this task has finally been embarked on, in accordance with our twentieth-century ideal of a medical science that is at once comprehensive, rational, and reliable in the highest degree, then we will have achieved the optimum.

Notes

I. CHINESE AND WESTERN MEDICINE

1. Meyer-Steineg and Sudhoff, *Illustrierte Geschichte der Medizin,* 5th ed., p. 30.
2. Jores, *Die Medizin in der Krise unserer Zeit,* p. 38.
3. Meyer-Steineg and Sudhoff, op. cit., p. 320.
4. Helberger, "Ziele und Ergebnisse der Gesundheitspolitik," p. 686.
5. Schaefer, *Die Medizin heute,* p. 113.
6. Jores, op. cit., p. 54.
7. Helberger, op. cit., p. 691.
8. Ibid., p. 690.
9. Noelle-Neumann (ed.), *Allensbacher Jahrbuch der Demoskopie 1976,* p. 180. To the question "By and large, how would you characterize your usual state of health?" 18 percent of respondents answered "Very good," 41 percent "Rather good," 35 percent "Fair," 5 percent "Rather bad," and 1 percent "Very bad."
10. Jores, op. cit., p. 26f.
11. According to Berlin neurologist Roland Schiffter, *"Akupunktur aus der Sicht eines kritischen Neurologen"* in *Akupunktur,* January 1974.
12. *Süddeutsche Zeitung,* July 30, 1977.
13. von Uexküll, "An den Grenzen der Medizin," p. 100.
14. From the Greek *iatros* (doctor) and *genesis* (origin, cause).
15. Jores, op. cit., p. 58.
16. Ibid., p. 54.
17. Whorf, *Language, Thought and Reality,* pp. 213–14.
18. Ibid., p. 252.
19. Ibid., pp. 27, 246.
20. Kuhn, *The Structure of Scientific Revolutions,* p. 24. Modern medical science can certainly be included among the "normal sciences," as that term is defined by Kuhn (*Structure,* p. 14).
21. Whorf, op. cit., p. 240.
22. Whorf, op. cit., pp. 211–20.
23. Stegmüller, *Theorie und Erfahrung,* p. 8.

292   24. Bichat quoted in Meyer-Steineg and Sudhoff, *Illustrierte Geschichte der Medizin*, p. 229.
   25. von Weizsäcker, "Der Arzt und der Kranke," 1927.
   26. Whorf, op. cit., p. 221.
   27. C. G. Jung, introduction to Richard Wilhelm's translation of *The Secret of the Golden Flower* (*Das Geheimnis der Goldenen Blüte*), p. 74.
   28. Idem.
   29. See Part VII, the chapter titled "Great Doctors and the Classical Texts," for a more complete discussion of the classical medical literature.
   30. Dr. A. Tartarinoff, who accompanied a Tsarist diplomatic mission to Peking c. 1850, was struck by the fact that "there is no trace of anatomical knowledge in all Chinese medicine" or "such as there is is so feeble as to be beneath notice." "Notes on the Use of Hydropathy and Pain-killers in China," which appeared in a collection titled *Arbeiten der Kaiserlichen Russischen Gesandtschaft zu Peking über China, sein Volk, seine Religion, seinen Institutionen, socialen Verhältnisse*, edited by Drs. Carl Abel and F. A. Mecklenburg, Berlin 1858.
   31. Wittgenstein, *Philosophische Untersuchungen 43*, p. 311.
   32. Granet, *La pensée chinoise* (German version, *Das chinesische Denken*, tr. Porkert, p. 87).
   33. Nogier, "Über die Akupunktur der Ohrmuschel" 1957.
   34. A technical term that literally means "heat"; see p. 173 for a more detailed explanation.
   35. Based on Franz Hübotter's translation in "Zwei berühmte chinesische Ärzte des Altertums, Chouen Yu-I und Hoa T'ouo," p. 19.
   36. Hübotter, op. cit., p. 15.
   37. Tartarinoff, loc. cit.

II. FUNDAMENTALS

   1. This chapter is entitled "Great Treatise on the Phenomena Corresponding to *Yang* and *Yin*." See p. 240 for more about the *Suwen* itself.

III. ORBISICONOGRAPHY

   1. N. R. Hanson, *Patterns of Discovery*. A detailed discussion of the problematical character of scientific "objectivity" may also be found in Wolfgang Stegmüller's *Theorie und Erfahrung*, particularly Part II, "Theorienstrukturen und Theoriendynamik."
   2. The arterial pathways (*sinarteriae*) are generally (and we believe not very aptly) referred to as "meridians" in most Western books about Chinese medicine.
   3. Hübotter, *Die chinesische Medizin*, p. 316.
   4. Quoted in Porkert, *Die theoretischen Grundlagen der chinesischen Medizin*, p. 133.

IV. SINARTERIOLOGY

1. Manaka and Urquhart, *The Layman's Guide to Acupuncture*, p. 129ff.
2. For a more detailed discussion of the reticular pathways (*sinarteriae reticulares*), see Porkert, *Die theoretischen Grundlagen der chinesischen Medizin*, p. 150ff.
3. See, e.g., the two books just mentioned, in addition to "An Outline of Chinese Acupuncture," a publication of the Peking Academy for Traditional Chinese Medicine (Beijing: Foreign Language Press, 1975). The literature on acupuncture in Western languages frequently contains useful illustrations depicting the courses of the arterial pathways and the locations of the impulse points, but it is not very satisfactory from the standpoint of Chinese medical theory. These works generally only mention the clinical indications for particular *foramina* (i.e., the illnesses that may be treated by stimulating these points) without describing the precise functional effects that such a procedure is likely to have.

V. DIAGNOSIS

1. Ernst Mayr, *Principles of Systematic Zoology*, p. 13.
2. Chapter 62/547 of the *Suwen*, quoted in Porkert, *Lehrbuch der chinesischen Diagnostik*, p. 35.
3. Chapter 17/178, quoted in Porkert, loc. cit.
4. *Shanghan Zabinglun*, Chapter 1, quoted in Porkert, op. cit., p. 36.
5. For further particulars see Porkert, op. cit., p. 45.
6. Chapter 4 of the *Suwen*.
7. Porkert, loc. cit.
8. This doctrine was espoused by the school of Todo Yoshimasu; see Otsuka, *Kanpo, Geschichte, Theorie und Praxis der Chinesisch-Japonischen Traditionellen Medizin*.
9. Bachmann, *Die Akupunktur—eine Ordnungstherapie*, 2nd ed., p. 68ff.

VI. THERAPY

1. Chapter 13 of *The Yellow Prince's Classic*.
2. For example, Porkert, *Die klinische chinesische Pharmakologie*.
3. Cf. *Acta Medicinae Sinensis 1981*, Vols. 8 and 9; the observations of Professor Wolters, a West German chemist who visited the People's Republic on a fact-finding tour in 1978, are also quite interesting in this respect. He astonished the press on his return by reporting that a case of the flu that it would take ten days to cure by conventional Western means could be cured in only two days with traditional Chinese remedies (based on a scientific Chinese diagnosis). Professor Wolters, now employed by the pharmaceutical firm of Hoechst AG, does not have the reputation of being a particularly avid partisan of Chinese medicine as such.
4. Manaka, personal communication with the author.

294 VII. THE HISTORY OF CHINESE MEDICINE

1. Based on Hui Wen, "Acupuncture Anesthesia in Brain Surgery" in *Acupuncture Anesthesia.*
2. Quoted in *Acupuncture Anesthesia.*
3. Mao Zedong, "The United Front in Cultural Work," *Selected Works,* Vol. 3.
4. Quoted in Burchett and Alley, *China: The Quality of Life,* p. 229.
5. Horn, *Away with All Pests,* p. 87.
6. Idem.
7. *Huangdi Neijing*, Chapter 1.
8. *Idem.*
9. *Shanghan Zabinglun.*
10. Biography of Hua Tuo taken from Volume 920 of the *Great Imperial Encyclopedia* (tr. Porkert).
11. Quoted in Porkert, "Hua Tuo—ein chinesischer Chirurg im 2. Jahrhundert unserer Zeitrechnung," p. 527.
12. Ibid., p. 524.
13. Ibid., p. 521.
14. Ibid., p. 522ff.
15. Tartarinoff, op. cit., p. 423ff.
16. Quoted in Hartner, "Heilkunde im alten China," 1941–42.
17. *Acupuncture Anesthesia,* pp. 4–5.
18. "Akupunktur-Narkose nur Propagandalüge," *Frankfurter Allgemeine Zeitung,* November 5, 1980.
19. Whorf, op. cit., p. 209.

VIII. THE CURRENT SITUATION

1. Whorf, op. cit., p. 246.
2. Stegmüller, *Hauptströmungen der Gegenwartsphilosophie,* Vol. 2, p. 733.
3. Pfohl, "Vom Verlust akademischer Gesinnung," 1980.
4. Jores, op. cit., p. 54.

Selected Bibliography

THE methodical investigation of traditional Chinese medicine with the intent of eventually putting its resources at the disposal of the international scientific community has been under way for little more than two decades, even in East Asia. Before that, Chinese medicine was dismissed either as a "historical relic" or as a miscellaneous collection of empirical odds and ends that could be profitably exploited or rationally accounted for only with the aid of Western scientific principles. This explains the relative scarcity of useful secondary sources in this field, particularly in Western languages; it also explains why the existing professional societies are primarily concerned with the exchange of technical information (*"Rezeptakupunktur,"* "acupuncture by the numbers") rather than exploring more fundamental methodological questions in the broader context of Chinese scientific theory.

The picture of Chinese medicine that has been presented here is based essentially on the original sources; we hope we have not given the impression, however (as the Chinese themselves are sometimes wont to do) that the classic medical texts still represent the definitive and inexhaustible source of medical knowledge and technical expertise that they did a thousand years ago. It would be accurate to say that these works presented for the first time, in their essential form, a number of scientific theories that are no less valid today; it would not be correct to say that the scientific system that is embodied in these works completely corresponds to Chinese medical science in its present state or that it is adequate to meet the demands of the present day. This system has been progressively refined and tested, revised and developed until it has reached a level of maturity that is sufficient to justify the claims that have been made for it in this book. (Thus it is quite unlikely that even a student with the best possible background in medicine and philology could hope to recapitulate this process in a single lifetime by starting

296   afresh with the ancient texts and attempting to achieve a real mastery of the system, as it is presently constituted, on that basis alone.)

In fact, such a feat has become possible only in recent years, thanks largely to the vast project (that began during the 1950s) of cataloging and synthesizing the scattered remnants of Chinese medicine. Foremost among the names that deserve to be mentioned in this connection is of course the magisterial *General Presentation of Chinese Medicine* (*Zhong-yixue Gailun*), prepared by the Nanking Academy for Traditional Chinese Medicine. The first edition, of 1958, was published by Renmin Weisheng Chubanshe, Beijing (530 pages). A second, revised edition appeared in the following year, in which the discussion of a number of important topics (notably of *phase dynamics,* the aspect of Chinese medicine that deals with the relationship between cyclical, external events such as the cycle of the seasons, and diagnostic and therapeutic medicine) was greatly expanded. The first edition was reprinted during the 1970s by Yiyao Weisheng Chubanshe, a Hong Kong publishing house, largely for the benefit of the overseas Chinese community. (As mentioned earlier, these first two editions of the *Zhongyixue* managed to present the subject expertly and comprehensively without recourse to Western terminology or Western conceptual models.)

The demand for textbooks (in modern colloquial Chinese) led to a conference of representatives of all the academies for traditional medicine in Shanghai in 1963, at which it was decided to publish a series of commentaries on classical texts and monographs on numerous subspecialties within the realm of Chinese medicine. Twenty-six titles appeared in all, collectively known as *Zhongyixue jiaocai* (*Teaching Materials on Traditional Chinese Medicine*), all published by the Shanghai Science and Technology Press (Shanghai Kexaejishu Chubanshe). An excellent textbook on acu-moxa-therapy prepared by the Shanghai Academy for Traditional Chinese Medicine (Shanghai Zhonoyi Xueyuan) was supplanted in 1974 by a truly monumental work on the same subject, also compiled by the Shanghai Academy and simply titled *Zhenjiuxue* (*Acu-Moxa-Therapy*).

Finally, a second series of monographs appeared during the 1970s. The original series, though naturally more comprehensive than the one-volume *General Presentation* of 1958, was not as authoritative and lacked the terminological rigor of the earlier work; similarly, this "third generation" of text materials that appeared during the early 1970s had become increasingly dependent on Western terminology and a Western theoretical frame of reference and thus was comparatively lacking in scientific value.

Acupuncture Anesthesia. Beijing, 1972.

Bachmann, Gerhard. *Die Akupunktur—eine Ordnungstherapie,* 2 vols., 2nd ed. Heidelberg, 1976.

Burchett, Wilfred, and Alley, Rewy. *China, The Quality of Life.* Baltimore, 1976.

Fu Wei-kang. *The Story of Chinese Acupuncture and Moxibustion.* Peking, 1975.

Granet, Marcel. *La pensée chinoise.* Paris, 1934 (German tr. Porkert, München, 1963).

Hanson, N. R. *Patterns of Discovery.* Cambridge, 1958.

Hartner, Willy. "Heilkunde im alten China," *Sinica.* Frankfurt, 1941–42.

Helberger, Christof. "Ziele und Ergebnisse der Gesundheitspolitik" in Wolfgang Zapf (ed.), *Lebensbedingungen in der Bundesrepublik, Sozialer Wandel und Wohlfahrtsentwicklung.* Frankfurt, 1977.

Hoangdi neijing suwen yishi. Shanghai, 1959 (also *Lingshu baihuajie,* Beijing, 1963). Other renderings of *The Yellow Prince's Classic* into modern colloquial Chinese (with commentary) have appeared since the 1950s. The existing versions in French (by Chamfrault and Nguyen Van Nghi) and English (Ilza Veith, *The Yellow Emperor's Classic of Internal Medicine*) may be approached as curiosities of the history of medicine, but though they may convey the requisite whiff of *couleur locale,* the translators have failed to adopt an unambiguous normative terminology, which makes both of these works relatively useless for purposes of scientific reconstruction.

Horn, Joshua S. *Away with All Pests, An English Surgeon in People's China.* London, 1972.

Hübotter, Franz. *Die chinesische Medizin.* Leipzig, 1929.

———. "Berühmte chinesische Ärzte" in *Archiv für Geschichte der Medizin,* 7. Band. Leipzig, 1914.

———. "Zwei berühmte chinesische Ärzte des Altertums: Chouen Yu-J und Hoa T'ouo" in *Mitteilungen der Deutschen Gesellschaft für Natur und Volkerkunde Ostasiens.* Band XXI, Teil A. Tokyo, 1926.

298 Jores, Arthur. *Die Medizin in der Krise unserer Zeit.* Bern, 1961.

Jung, C. G. Introduction to *Das Geheimnis der Goldenen Blüte.* (tr. Richard Wilhelm). Zurich, 1928, 1948 (*The Secret of the Golden Flower,* tr. Cary Baynes). New York, 1962.

Kleinmann, Arthur; Kunstader, Peter; and Alexander, E. Russell. *Medicine in Chinese Culture: Comparative Studies of Health Care in Chinese and Other Societies.* Washington, 1974.

Kuhn, Thomas S. *The Structure of Scientific Revolutions.* Chicago, 1962.

Leslie, Charles (ed.) *Asian Medical Systems: A Comparative Study.* Berkeley, 1976.

Manaka, Yoshio, and Urquhart, Ian A. *The Layman's Guide to Acupuncture.* New York, 1972.

Mayr, Ernst. *Principles of Systematic Zoology.* New York, 1969.

Meyer-Steineg, Th., and Sudhoff, K. *Illustrierte Geschichte der Medizin.* Stuttgart, 1965.

Mojing ("The Pulse Classic") (tr. Franz Hübotter) in *Die chinesische Medizin im 20. Jahrhundert und ihr historischer Werdegang,* pp. 239–72.

Noelle-Neumann, Elisabeth (ed.) *Allenbacher Jahrbuch der Demoskopie 1976.* Wien, 1976.

Nogier, Paul. "Über die Akupunktur der Ohrmuschel," *Deutsche Zeitschrift für Akupunktur,* Nr. 3–4, 5–6, 7–8, 1957.

Otsuka, Keisetu. *Kanpo, Geschichte, Theorie und Praxis der Chinesisch-Japonischen Traditionellen Medizin.* Tokyo, 1976.

Pfohl, Gerhard, "Vom Verlust akademischer Gesinnung." Festvortrag des Festaktes *20 Jahre Forschungszentrum Neuherberg.* December 10, 1980. Manuskript der Gesellschaft fur Strahlen- und Umweltforschung.

Rothschuh, Karl E. (ed.), *Was ist Krankheit?* Darmstadt, 1975.

Schaefer, Hans. *Die Medizin heute.* München, 1963.

Schiffter, Roland, "Akupunktur aus der Sicht eines kritischen Neurologen," *Akupunktur,* 1/74.

Stegmüller, Wolfgang. *Hauptströmungen der Gegenwartsphilosophie,* Vol. II. Stuttgart, 1979.

———. *Theories und Erfahrung.* Berlin, 1973.

Tartarinoff, A. "Bemerkungen uber die Anwendung schmerzstillender Mittel bei den Operationen und uber die Hydropathie in China" in Carl Abel and F. A. Mecklenburg (eds.), *Arbeiten der Kaiserlich Russischen Gesandtschaft zu Peking* ... Berlin, 1858.

Uexküll, Thure von. "An den Grenzen der Medizin" in Heinrich Nussbaum (ed.), *Die verordnete Krankheit.* Frankfurt, 1977.

Weizsacker, Viktor von. "Der Arzt und der Kranke" (1927) in Karl E. Rothschuh (ed.), *Was ist Krankheit?* Darmstadt, 1975.

Whorf, Benjamin Lee. *Language, Thought and Reality,* John B. Carroll, ed. Cambridge, Mass., 1956.

Wittgenstein, Ludwig. *Philosophische Untersuchungen 43.* Frankfurt, 1963.

Zhongyixue Gailun. Nanking Academy of Traditional Chinese Medicine. 299
Renmin Weisheng Chubanshe. Beijing, 1958; 2nd ed., 1959; 1st rev. ed.,
1970, Yiyao Weisheng Chubanshe. Hong Kong, 1970.

WORKS BY MANFRED PORKERT

Die theoretischen Grundlagen der chinesischen Medizin. Wiesbaden, 1973. (*The
Theoretical Foundations of Chinese Medicine*. Cambridge, Mass. 1978.)

Lehrbuch der chinesischen Diagnostik. Heidelberg, 1976. (*The Essentials of Chinese
Diagnostics*, AMS Monographs, in preparation.)

Die klinische chinesische Pharmakologie. Heidelberg, 1978.

"Die Heilung von Magen- und Darmgeschwüren durch ch'i-Übungen," *Basler
Nachrichten*, December 17, 1960.

"Chinas Medizin heute," *Handelsblatt*, October 21, 1960.

"Das neue Lehrbuch der chinesischen Medizin," *Handelsblatt*, November 12,
1960.

"Hua T'uo—ein chinesischer Chirurg im 2. Jahrhundert unserer Zeitrechnung"
in *Die Grossen der Welt* (Kindler Verlag: Zurich, 1971).

"Die elementaren Fragen in Inneren Klassiker des Gelben Fursten (*Huang-ti
Nei-ching Su-wen*)—Über den ältesten Klassiker der chinesischen Medizin," *Basler Nachrichten*, May 24, 1963.

"The Intellectual and Social Impulses Behind the Evolution of Chinese
Medicine" in *Wenner Gren Symposium*, 53, 1971.

"Die Akupunktur und der Schmerz," *TR-Verlagsunion*, München 1974.

"On the Dilemma of Present-Day Interpretations of Chinese Medicine and on
the Ways to Overcome This Dilemma," *NIH Conference Proceedings*, 1974.

"Die andere, die chinesische Medizin," *Süddeutsche Zeitung*, July 15, 1974, and
Münchener Ärztliche Anzeigen, 17/1975

"Die energetische Terminologie in den chinesischen Medizinklassikern," *Sino-
logica*, 2/1965.

"Die historischen und methodischen Bedingungen der chinesischen Medizin,"
München, 1975.

"Die wissenschaftliche Ort der Akupunktur." *Münchener Medizinische Wochen-
schrift*, April 2, 1976.

"Die sachlichen Pramissen fur eine wissenschaftliche Diskussion der Akupunktur," *Deutsche Ärzteblatt*, April 29, 1976.

"Die verschiedenen Fassungen der 'Allgemeinen Darstellung der Chinesischen
Medizin' (*Chung-I-Hsueh Kai-lun*) als Beispiel für den Wandel des
wissenschaftlichen Verständnisses der traditionellen Medizin in der
Volksrepublik China" in *Festschrift für Herbert Franke*. Wiesbaden.

Index